Color Atlas
of Soft Tissue
Tumors

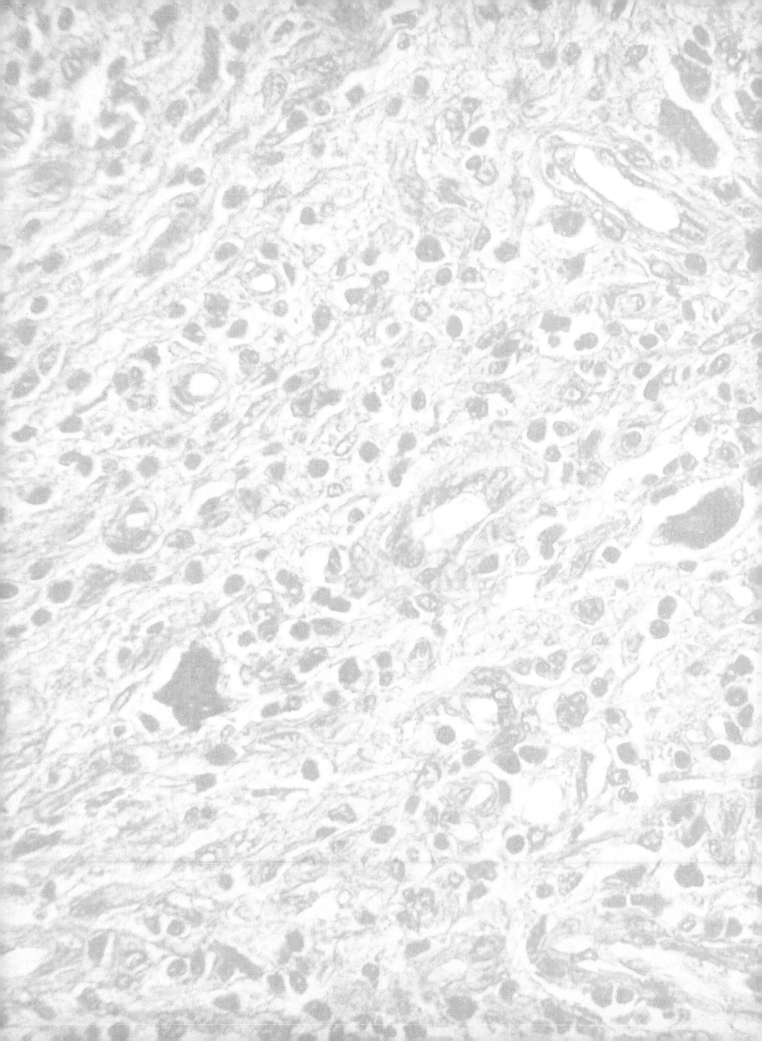

Color Atlas of Soft Tissue Tumors

Jeanne M. Meis-Kindblom, M.D.
Professor of Pathology,
University of Gothenburg
Gothenburg, Sweden
Former Chair, Department of Soft Tissue Pathology
Armed Forces Institute of Pathology
Washington, DC

Franz M. Enzinger, M.D.
Former Chair, Department of Soft Tissue Pathology
Armed Forces Institute of Pathology
Washington, DC

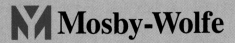 Mosby-Wolfe

St. Louis Baltimore Boston Carlsbad Chicago Naples New York Philadelphia Portland
London Madrid Mexico City Singapore Sydney Tokyo Toronto Wiesbaden

Mosby-Wolfe

Dedicated to Publishing Excellence

A Times Mirror Company

Publisher: Anne S. Patterson
Senior Managing Editor: Lynne Gery
Project Manager: Linda Clarke
Senior Production Editor: Vicki Hoenigke
Design Manager: Nancy McDonald
Electronic Composition Artist: Christine H. Poullain
Manufacturing Supervisor: Linda Ierardi

Printed in the United States of America
Composition by Mosby Electronic Production, Philadelphia
Printing/binding by Rand McNally Book Services

Mosby–Year Book, Inc.
11830 Westline Industrial Drive
St. Louis, MO 63146

Library of Congress Cataloging-in-Publication Data

Meis-Kindblom, Jeanne, M.
    Color atlas of soft tissue tumors / Jeanne M. Meis-Kindblom, Franz M. Enzinger
      p.   cm.
  Includes index.
  ISBN 0-8151-5895-5 (alk. paper)
  1. Soft tissue tumors—Atlases. I. Enzinger, Franz M. II. Title.
  [DNLM: 1. Soft Tissue Neoplasms—pathology—atlases. WD 375
M515c   1996]
RC280.S66M45   1996
616.99'2—dc20
DNLM/DLC
for Library of Congress
                                         95-9592
                                          CIP

96 97 98 99 / 9 8 7 6 5 4 3 2 1

Preface

The diagnosis of soft tissue tumors may be difficult for several reasons. One reason is that soft tissue tumors are relatively rare. Therefore, most pathologists are not exposed to many soft tissue lesions during their training and only occasionally encounter them in the practice of surgical pathology. Another reason is that many soft tissue tumors have overlapping histologic appearances, rendering the distinction between reactive versus neoplastic and benign versus malignant more difficult. The clinical implications of a benign versus a malignant process are dramatic in terms of the type and extent of surgery performed and whether the patient will receive chemotherapy or radiotherapy. The use of ancillary techniques has increased insight into the biology of soft tissue tumors and has provided tools for greater diagnostic accuracy, yet the foundation of these newer techniques rests upon the correct histologic diagnosis. Moreover, in an era where economic restraints are having an increasing impact on medical practice, accurate light microscopy remains the simplest, fastest, and most economic method of diagnosis.

The purpose of this atlas is to facilitate the diagnosis of soft tissue tumors by illustrating a broad array of soft tissue tumors. Typical and less common appearances are shown. Each diagnosis is presented in the same format. First, a summary of the tumor is given in terms of disease presentation, age groups commonly affected, behavior, and prognosis. This is followed by a checklist of diagnostic features, proceeding from architectural to cytologic features to a description of the matrix to secondary tumor features. Another checklist of differential diagnoses follows. A variety of pictures illustrate the morphologic spectrum seen within each diagnostic category with captions that comment upon specific features in the illustrations. The illustrations have been culled from a large collection of soft tissue photos gathered over a number of years from consultation cases and thus represent a condensation of many years of experience in the diagnosis of soft tissue tumors.

This book could be used alone or as a supplement to other references on soft tissue tumors. Since surgical pathology (among several other medical specialties) requires visual recognition of a variety of patterns, a color atlas demonstrating the numerous facets and various diagnostic entities seems to be one of the best ways to become familiar with soft tissue tumors, particularly if one does not have the opportunity to do it firsthand. An atlas can also reinforce and refresh one's visual memory. The condensed text is useful for rapidly looking up the salient diagnostic features, and the numerous illustrations demonstrate most of the patterns seen in soft tissue tumors. This atlas, it is hoped, will be stimulating, educational, and a useful adjunct in the diagnosis and treatment of soft tissue tumors for our colleagues in the medical profession.

JEANNE M. MEIS-KINDBLOM, M.D.

FRANZ M. ENZINGER, M.D.

Contents

Color Atlas
of Soft Tissue
Tumors

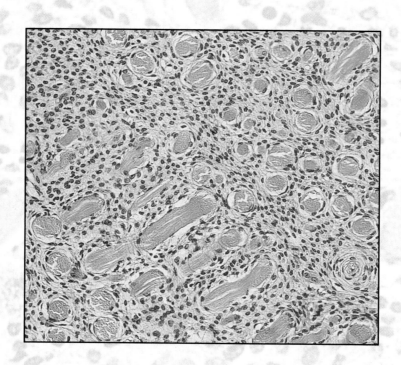

Chapter 1

Fibrous Tissue Tumors

BENIGN
Fibroma

Fibroma is a general term that most commonly refers to the polypoid skin lesions fibroma durum and fibroma molle, which contain variable amounts of fibrous connective tissue and fat, respectively. Such lesions are probably reactive.

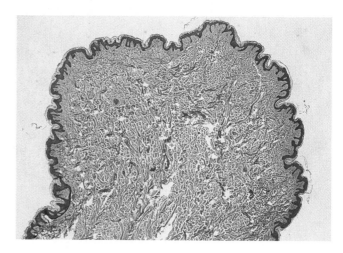

Fig. 1-1 Typical example of fibroma durum of skin with a polypoid configuration and prominent collagenous component in the dermis.

Nodular Fasciitis

Nodular fasciitis is the most frequently encountered pseudosarcomatous proliferation of fibrous tissue. It is believed to be reactive in nature and occurs most frequently in the upper extremities of patients in the third and fourth decades of life. It usually involves the subcutis, but intramuscular forms also occur. Variants include intravascular fasciitis, cranial fasciits, and ossifying (parosteal) fasciitis. **Intravascular fasciitis** involves small to medium arteries and veins and occurs primarily in children and young adults. **Cranial fasciitis** usually affects infants less than 1 year of age and involves the scalp and skull. **Ossifying fasciitis,** which occurs in a periosteal location, is similar to myositis ossificans but lacks its zonal pattern or organization.

MICROSCOPIC FEATURES

- Well-circumscribed or stellate configuration
- Uniform (myo)fibroblasts with bland cytologic features
- Haphazard, whorled, or broad storiform pattern
- Variable amount of myxoid matrix imparting a "feathered" appearance
- Microcysts and macrocysts
- Keloid-like strands of collagen
- Lymphocytes
- Extravasated red blood cells
- Variable numbers of multinucleated giant cells

DIFFERENTIAL DIAGNOSIS

- Myxoma
- Fibrous histiocytoma
- Fibromatosis
- Fibrosarcoma
- Kaposi's sarcoma
- Leiomyosarcoma
- Myxoid malignant fibrous histiocytoma

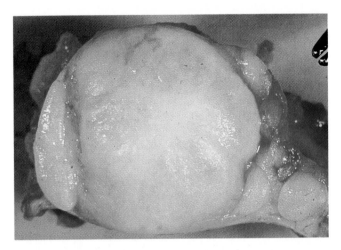

Fig. 1-2 Cut section of subcutaneous nodular fasciitis demonstrating circumscription and myxoid cut surface of lesion.

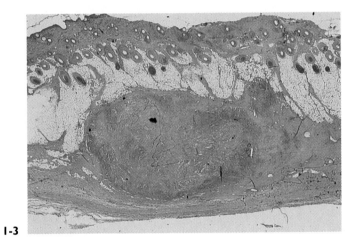

1-3

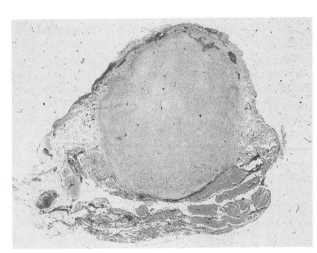

1-4

Figs. 1-3 and 1-4 Well-circumscribed examples of nodular fasciitis in the subcutis.

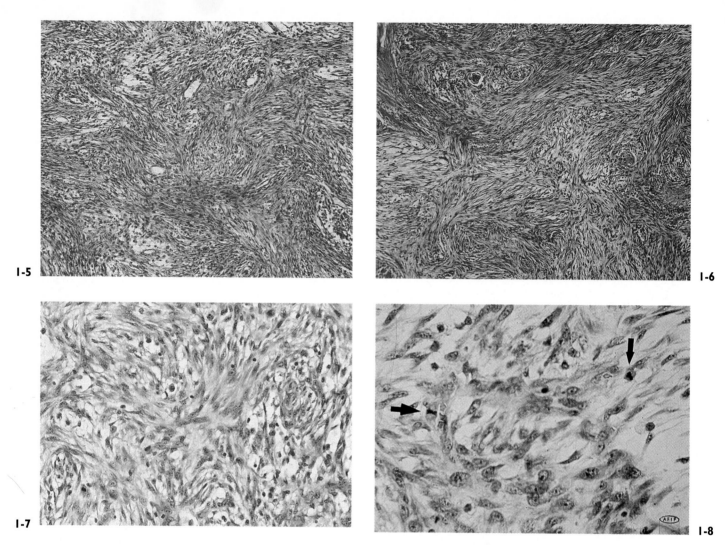

1-5

1-6

1-7

1-8

Figs. 1-5 through 1-16 Typical examples of nodular fasciitis with a variable amount of myxoid matrix and small cysts. Note the broad, whorled to storiform pattern, the cytologically bland nuclear features, and the elongated, basophilic cytoplasmic processes of the myofibroblasts. A brisk mitotic rate is not uncommon. The cells are fuchsinophilic with the trichrome stain (Fig. 1-16).

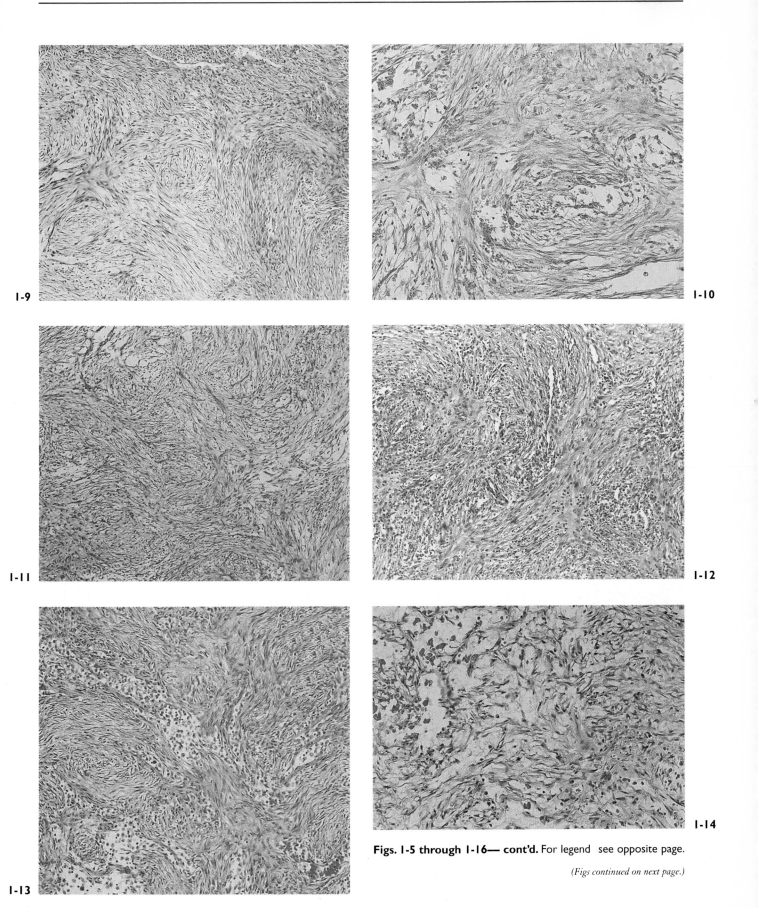

1-9

1-10

1-11

1-12

1-13

1-14

Figs. 1-5 through 1-16— cont'd. For legend see opposite page.

(Figs continued on next page.)

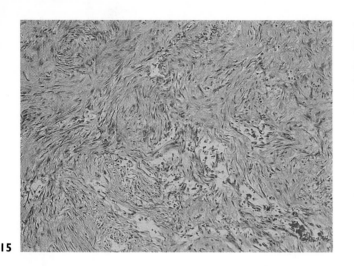

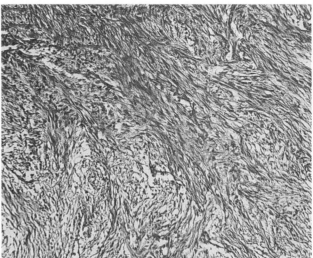

1-15

1-16

Figs. 1-5 through 1-16— cont'd. For legend, see page 4.

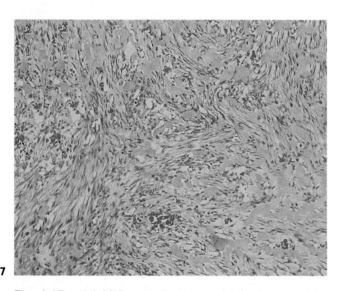

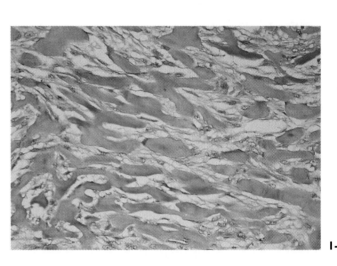

1-17

1-18

Figs. 1-17 and 1-18 Broad refractile strands of collagen reminiscent of those seen in a keloid are a frequent feature of nodular fasciitis, mostly in lesions that have been present for several weeks or months.

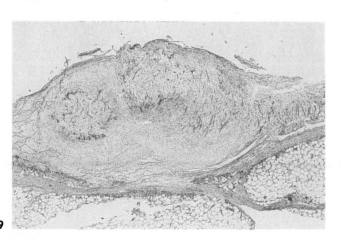

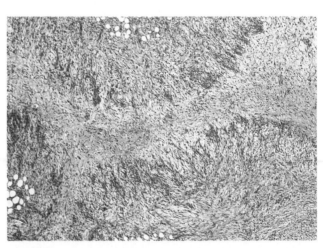

1-19

1-20

Figs. 1-19 and 1-20 Numerous, delicate small vessels may be seen in nodular fasciitis, closely resembling granulation tissue.

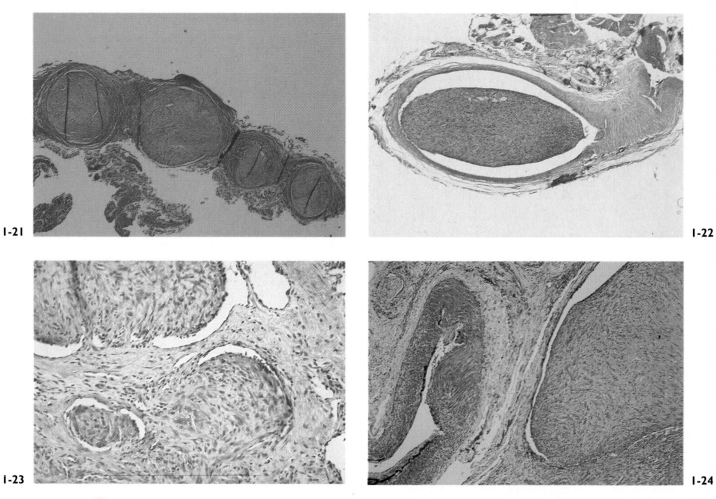

1-21

1-22

1-23

1-24

Figs. 1-21 through 1-24 Typical examples of intravascular fasciitis demonstrating intravascular growth that frequently results in a multi-nodular configuration or a polypoid intraluminal appearance (Movat stain, Fig. 1-24).

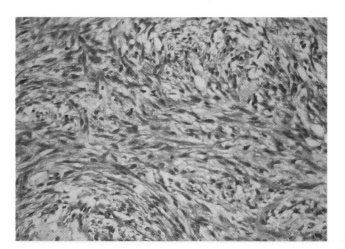

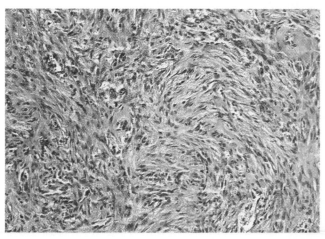

Fig. 1-25 The myofibroblastic proliferation of intravascular fasciitis is indistinguishable from that of nodular fasciitis.

Fig. 1-26 An example of cranial fasciitis. Note the close resemblance to nodular fasciitis.

Proliferative Fasciitis

Proliferative fasciitis, another pseudosarcomatous myofibroblastic proliferation, is much less common than nodular fasciitis. Although it occurs primarily in adults, rare cases may occur in children. The proximal extremities are most frequently affected. This type of fasciitis mainly involves the interlobular fibrous tissue septa of the subcutis and therefore is less well demarcated than most cases of nodular fasciitis.

MICROSCOPIC FEATURES

- Irregular or stellate configuration
- Ganglion cell–like (myo)fibroblasts
- Spindled (myo)fibroblasts
- Myxoid to collagenized matrix (variable)
- Septal distribution

DIFFERENTIAL DIAGNOSIS

- Malignant fibrous histiocytoma
- Rhabdomyosarcoma
- Ganglioneuroblastoma

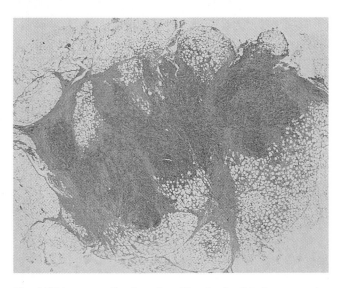

Fig. 1-27 Low magnification of proliferative fasciitis demonstrating growth along the fibrous septa of the subcutis.

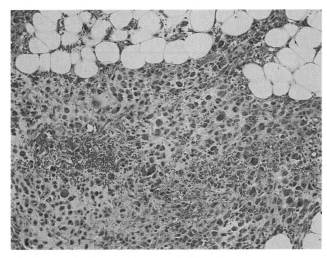

1-28

Figs. 1-28 through 1-33 Large, plump, ganglion cell-like (myo)fibroblasts are the hallmark of proliferative fasciitis. The close similarity to ganglion cells is attributable to the presence of large, vesicular nuclei containing prominent, inclusion-like basophilic to eosinophilic nucleoli, as well as abundant eosinophilic cytoplasm. These cells may be associated with occasional slender myofibroblasts and a variably myxoid to collagenous matrix. Intracytoplasmic collagen is frequently seen in proliferative fasciitis, as demonstrated by the presence of one or more prominent eosinophilic cytoplasmic inclusions (Fig. 1-33).

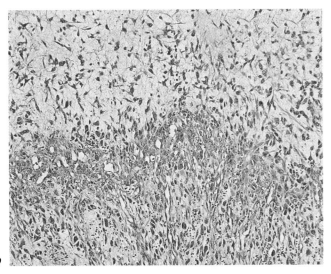

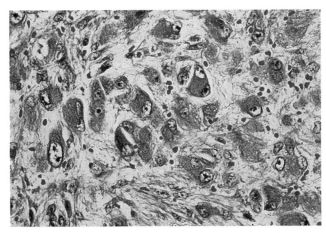

1-29

1-30

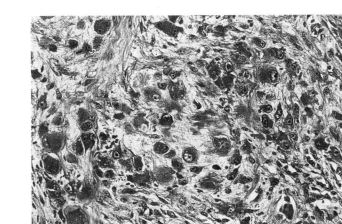

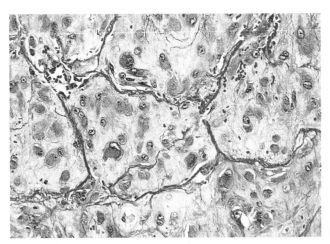

1-31

1-32

Figs. 1-28 through 1-33—cont'd. For legend, see opposite page.

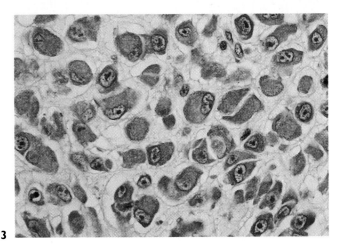

1-33

Proliferative Myositis

This type of myositis is the intramuscular counterpart of proliferative fasciitis. Like the other pseudosarcomatous myofibroblastic proliferations, it typically presents as a rapidly growing mass of short duration. Although it occurs most frequently in adults, children may also be affected. The trunk and the limb girdles are the usual sites. Typically the epimysium, perimysium, and endomysium are involved, which accounts for its ill-defined margins.

MICROSCOPIC FEATURES

- "Checkerboard" appearance (growth along fascial planes of muscle)
- Ganglion cell-like (myo)fibroblasts
- Spindled myofibroblasts
- Myxoid to collagenized matrix (variable)
- Atrophic skeletal muscle fibers

DIFFERENTIAL DIAGNOSIS

- Rhabdomyosarcoma
- Malignant fibrous histiocytoma
- Ganglioneuroblastoma
- Myxoid malignant fibrous histiocytoma

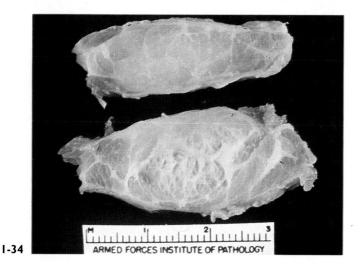

1-34

ARMED FORCES INSTITUTE OF PATHOLOGY

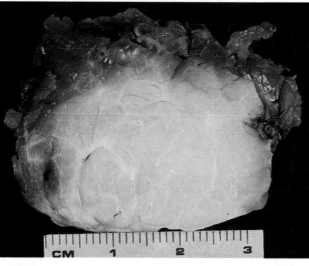

1-35

Figs. 1-34 and 1-35 Gross specimens of proliferative myositis demonstrating a vague multinodular appearance as a result of growth along the fascia and fibrous septa of the skeletal muscle.

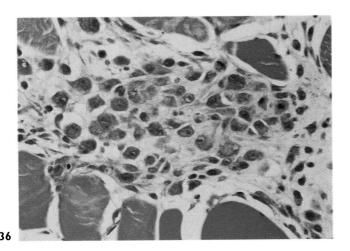

1-36

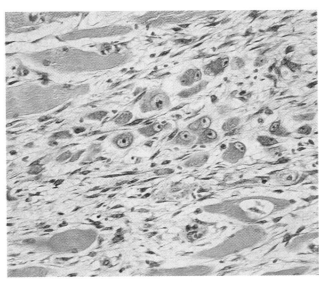

1-37

Figs. 1-36 and 1-37 Infiltration between skeletal muscle fibers is seen. The ganglion cell–like population of fibroblasts seen in proliferative myositis is virtually identical to that of proliferative fasciitis.

Atypical Decubital Fibroplasia

This pseudosarcomatous proliferation of myofibroblasts tends to occur over bony prominences (such as the sacrum or the ischial tuberosities) in immobilized or debilitated patients. Most patients are in their seventies or eighties. Atypical decubital fibroplasia bears a striking resemblance to proliferative fasciitis and in all likelihood is a largely unrecognized form of a deep pressure sore that involves the subcutis and occasionally the underlying musculature.

MICROSCOPIC FEATURES

- Ganglion cell–like (myo)fibroblasts
- Spindled (myo)fibroblasts
- Central fibrinous and myxoid zones
- Granulation tissue
- Acute inflammation (variable)

DIFFERENTIAL DIAGNOSIS

- Proliferative fasciitis and proliferative myositis
- Myxoid liposarcoma
- Myxoid malignant fibrous histiocytoma
- Chordoma

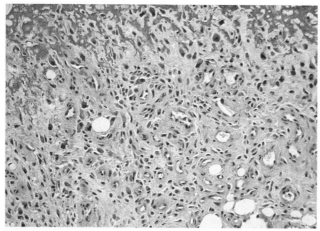

1-38

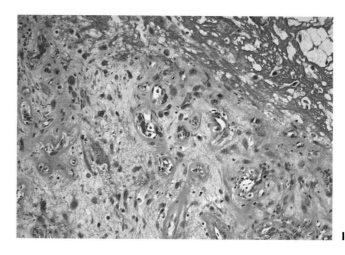

1-39

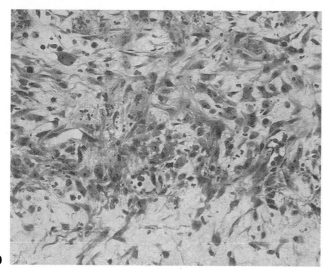

1-40

Figs. 1-38 through 1-40 Granulation tissue–like areas border fibrinous and myxoid zones containing enlarged, atypical, and degenerated fibroblasts; the latter resemble those seen in proliferative fasciitis and myositis.

Fibroma of Tendon Sheath

Fibroma of tendon sheath is a slow growing, reactive fibrous proliferation that usually involves the tendons of the hands or feet in adults. An early cellular phase may be seen in some cases, although most are hyalinized. Approximately 25% of cases recur locally.

MICROSCOPIC FEATURES

- Multilobular architecture
- Well-demarcated margins
- Attached to tendon
- Cleftlike spaces between lobules
- Densely collagenized-hyalinized matrix
- Scattered (myo)fibroblasts
- Chondro-osseous foci (rare)

DIFFERENTIAL DIAGNOSIS

- Fibrous histiocytoma
- Nodular fasciitis

- Fibromatosis
- Fibrosarcoma

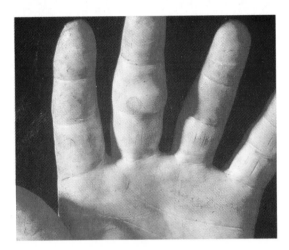

Fig. 1-41 Clinical example of fibroma of tendon sheath.

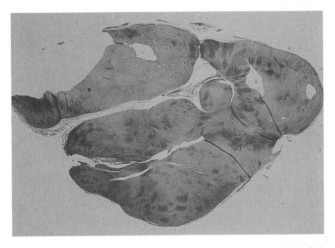

Fig. 1-42 Fibroma of tendon sheath at low magnification. The lesion is well circumscribed and demonstrates cleft-like spaces.

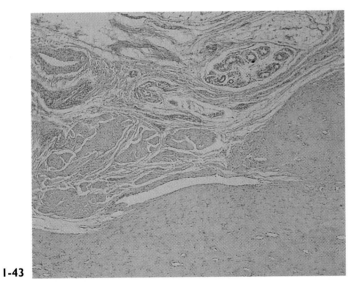

1-43

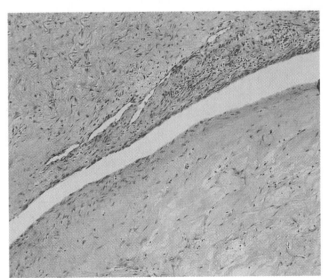

1-44

Figs. 1-43 through 1-46 Amorphous collagen, scattered bland fibroblasts, and occasional clefts simulating vessels are characteristic of fibroma of tendon sheath. Attachment to a tendon sheath may be seen.

(Figs continued on next page.)

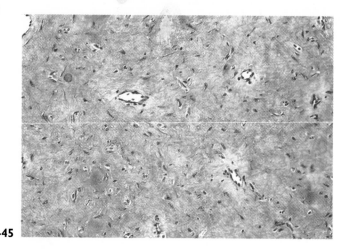

1-45

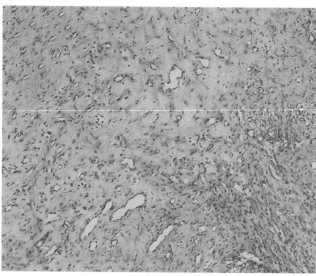

1-46

Figs. 1-43 through 1-46—cont'd. For legend, see page 13.

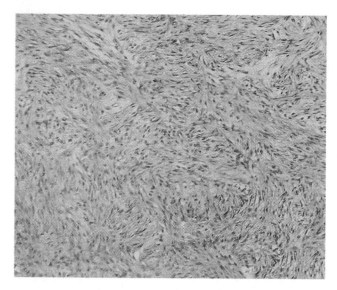

Fig. 1-47 A more cellular area of fibroma of tendon sheath. These areas are usually seen at the periphery of the lesion and may resemble nodular fasciitis or fibrous histiocytoma.

Elastofibroma

This reactive pseudotumor is composed of fibroblasts and myofibroblasts and is characterized by deranged elastic fibrillogenesis. Both the clinical and pathologic features of elastofibroma are quite distinctive. The elastofibroma is ill-defined, usually occurs in a subscapular location subjacent to the chest wall musculature, and is adherent to the underlying periosteum. There is a higher incidence reported in manual laborers, a potential genetic predisposition, and a higher incidence in females. Local recurrences are rare.

MICROSCOPIC FEATURES

- Ill-defined margins
- Predominantly hyalinized collagen
- Scant, scattered fibroblasts
- Thickened, serrated, deeply acidophilic elastic fibrils (diagnostic)
- Entrapped mature adipose tissue
- Myxoid matrix (rare)

DIFFERENTIAL DIAGNOSIS

- Fibrolipoma
- Fibromatosis

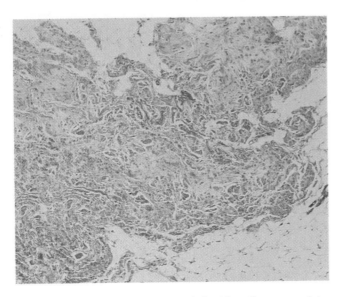

Fig. 1-48 Adipose tissue intermingled with collagen containing enlarged, eosinophilic elastic fibrils.

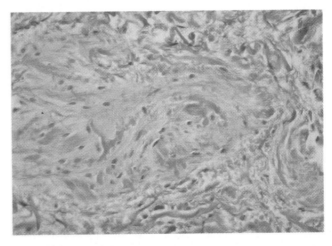

1-49

Figs. 1-49 through 1-52 The elastic fibrils of elastofibroma are markedly enlarged and serrated, resulting in a pipe cleaner–like appearance. The abnormal elastic fibrils are accentuated with special stains for collagen (Fig. 1-51) and elastic fibers (Fig. 1-52).

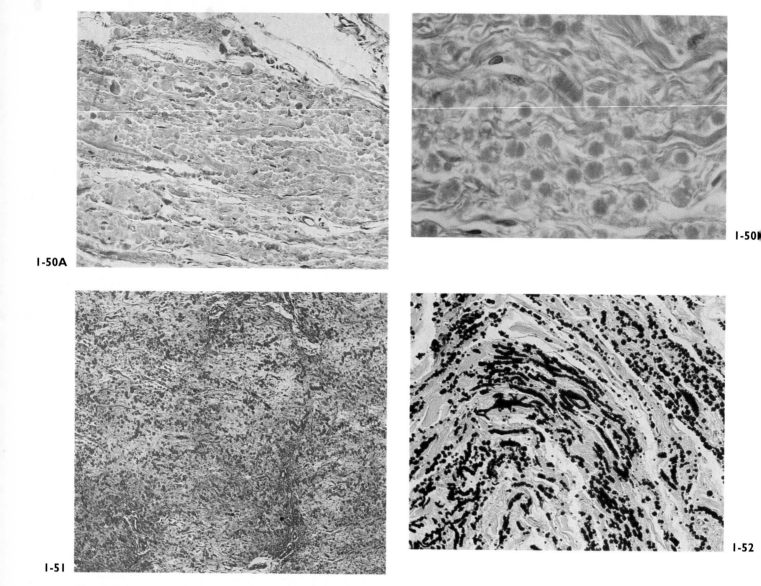

1-50A

1-50B

1-51

1-52

Figs. 1-49 through 1-52—cont'd. For legend, see page 15.

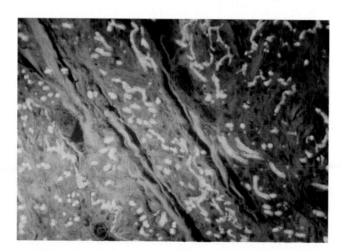

Fig. 1-53 The elastic fibrils of elastofibroma demonstrate autofluorescence.

Nuchal Fibroma

This paucicellular fibrous growth of the subcutis has a predilection for the interscapular and upper paraspinous regions of adults. It may recur if incompletely excised.

MICROSCOPIC FEATURES

- Paucicellular collagen bundles
- Mature fat
- Involvement of subcutis
- Calcification (variable)

DIFFERENTIAL DIAGNOSIS

- Fibrolipoma
- Fibromatosis

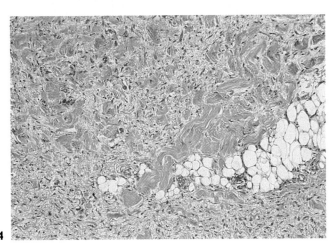
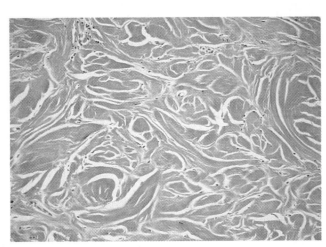

1-54   1-55

Figs. 1-54 and 1-55 Dense, fibrous connective tissue arranged in thick strands and amorphous sheets infiltrate the adjacent adipose tissue in nuchal fibroma.

Nasopharyngeal Angiofibroma

This richly vascular fibrous proliferation typically occurs in young males in the second decade. It generally presents as a lobulated, polypoid mass of the nasopharynx and paranasal sinuses that may cause nasal obstruction and profuse epistaxis. There is a high rate (up to 60%) of local recurrence.

MICROSCOPIC FEATURES

- Fibrous tissue of variable cellularity
- Hyalinization or myxoid change
- Prominent thin-walled vessels of variable caliber

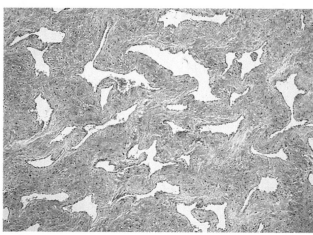
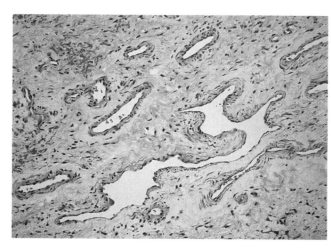

Figs. 1-56 and 1-57 A densely collagenous to fibromyxoid matrix surrounds numerous, dilated, ectatic vessels of nasopharyngeal angiofibroma.

Keloid

This reactive proliferation of fibrous connective tissue has a predilection for blacks and may also be familial. It tends to involve the upper body and usually occurs in adolescents or adults. It frequently follows trauma or surgery.

MICROSCOPIC FEATURES

- Glassy, hyalinized collagen fibers
- Haphazard arrangement of collagen fibers
- Myxoid matrix
- Calcification (variable)

DIFFERENTIAL DIAGNOSIS

- Hypertrophic scar
- Scleroderma (morphea)
- "Collagenoma"
- Fibromatosis

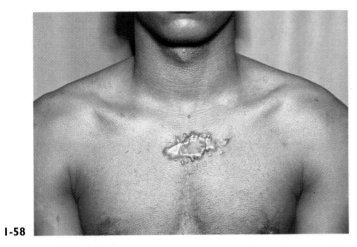

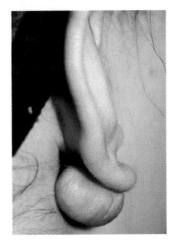

1-58

1-59

Figs. 1-58 and 1-59 Clinical examples of keloid at two characteristic locations.

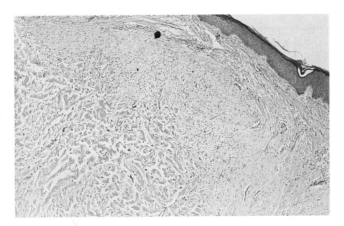

Fig. 1-60 Glassy, thickened, pale to deeply acidophilic bands of collagen and scattered fibroblasts are typical features of keloid.

FIBROUS TUMORS OF INFANCY AND CHILDHOOD

Fibrous Hamartoma of Infancy

This hamartomatous lesion is usually solitary and involves the dermis and subcutis of children who are usually younger than 1 year old. Roughly 20% of cases are congenital, and there is a slight male predominance. The axillary region, upper portions of the extremities, and inguinal regions are the most common sites. It does not occur in the hands and feet.

MICROSCOPIC FEATURES

- Ill-defined margins
- Organoid appearance
- Three tissue components (in varying proportions):
  1) Fibrous trabeculae or septa
  2) Myxoid foci containing small primitive stellate and spindled cells
  3) Mature fat
- Neurofibroma-like areas of fibrosis (variable)

DIFFERENTIAL DIAGNOSIS

- Infantile fibromatosis
- Infantile myofibromatosis
- Calcifying aponeurotic fibroma
- Infantile fibrosarcoma

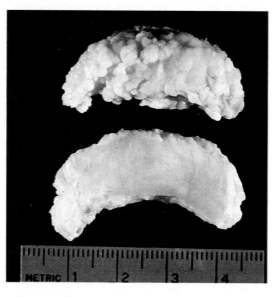

Fig. 1-61 Fat and fibrous bands are intermingled in this gross specimen of a fibrous hamartoma of infancy.

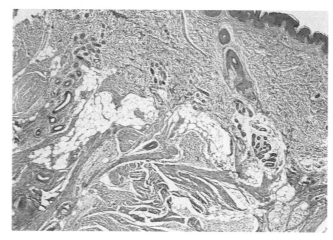

1-62

Figs. 1-62 through 1-69 Fibrous hamartoma of infancy is characteristically a superficial lesion. At low magnification, the fibrous and fatty elements are readily identified. In addition, there is a primitive mesenchymal element composed of spindled, bland cells that frequently are associated with a myxoid matrix. The fibrous component of fibrous hamartoma of infancy may at times resemble a keloid (Fig. 1-66). Trichrome and colloidal iron stains of fibrous hamartoma of infancy underscore the three components of this lesion (Figs. 1-67 through 1-69).

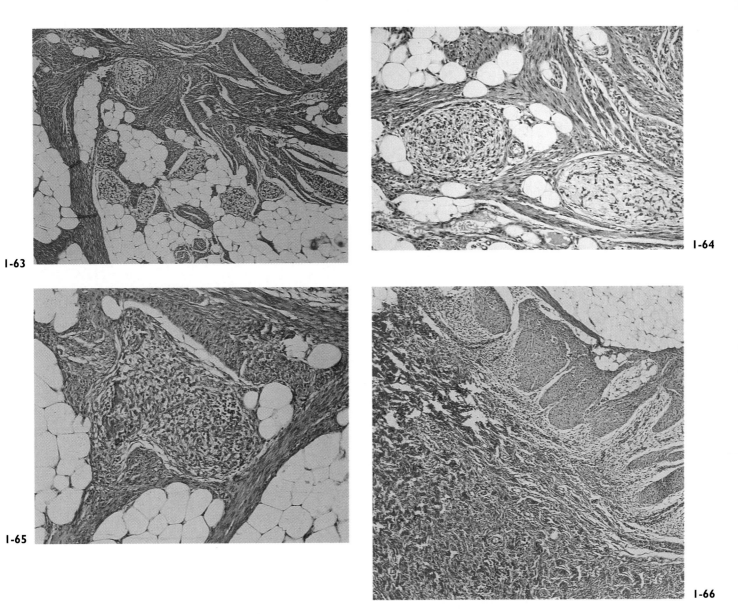

1-63

1-64

1-65

1-66

Figs. 1-62 through 1-69—cont'd. For legend, see opposite page.

(Figs continued on next page.)

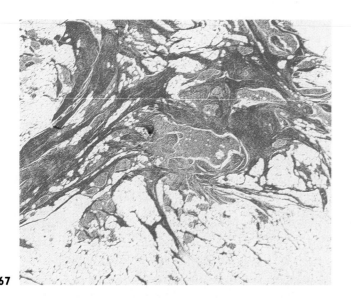

1-67

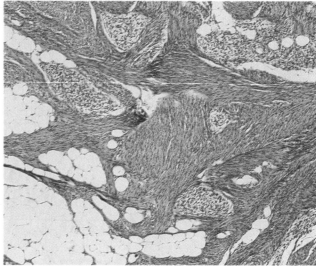

1-68

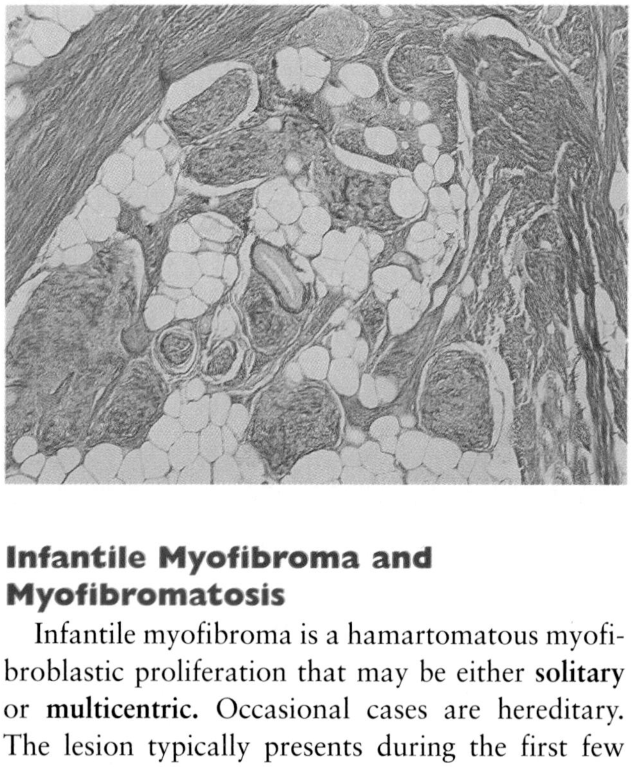

Figs. 1-62 through 1-69—cont'd. For legend, see page 20.

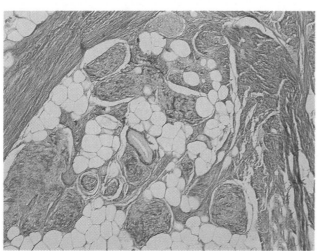

1-69

Infantile Myofibroma and Myofibromatosis

Infantile myofibroma is a hamartomatous myofibroblastic proliferation that may be either **solitary** or **multicentric.** Occasional cases are hereditary. The lesion typically presents during the first few weeks of life and may be congenital, although older children and adults may rarely be affected. The solitary form is located in the dermis, subcutis, or skeletal muscle and is more common than the multicentric form (myofibromatosis). Lesions of the latter type characteristically occur in the soft tissues, skeleton, lungs, heart, and gastrointestinal tract. The solitary form has a good prognosis and spontaneous regression is common. The multicentric form involving the viscera may lead to the patient's demise through secondary complications.

MICROSCOPIC FEATURES

- Zonal or multinodular pattern with "myoid" areas at periphery
- Leiomyoma-like short fascicles of myofibroblasts (peripherally)
- Necrosis (variable)

- Round-polygonal primitive cells around dilated vessels simulating hemangiopericytoma (central portion of lesion, variable)
- Calcification (variable)
- Intravascular growth (variable)

DIFFERENTIAL DIAGNOSIS

- Nodular (intravascular) fasciitis
- Leiomyoma
- Infantile fibromatosis

- Plexiform fibrohistiocytic tumor
- Neurofibromatosis
- Juvenile hyalin fibromatosis

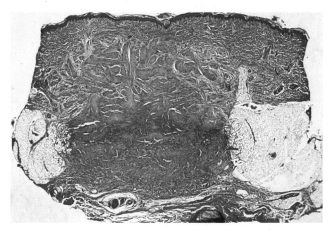

Fig. 1-70 A relatively well-circumscribed, infantile myofibroma of the skin involves the dermis and subcutis.

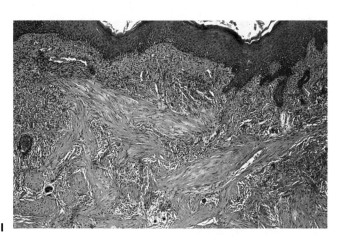

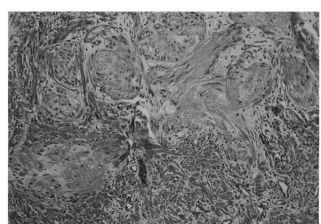

1-71

1-72

Figs. 1-71 through 1-74 These infantile myofibromas are less well defined. Note the arrangement of myfibroblasts into bundles that closely resemble smooth muscle in some portions of the lesion (trichrome stain, Fig. 1-73).

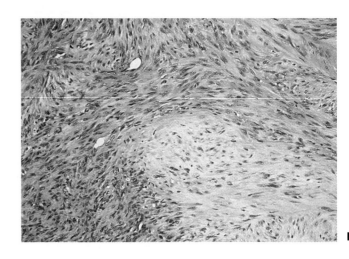

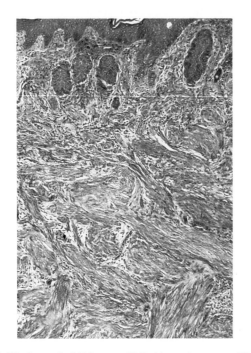

1-74

1-73

Figs. 1-71 through 1-74—cont'd For legend, see page 23.

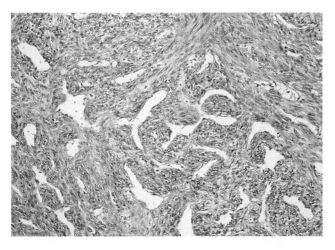

Fig. 1-75 Areas with a prominent hemangiopericytoma-like vascular pattern may be seen in the central portions of some infantile myofibromas.

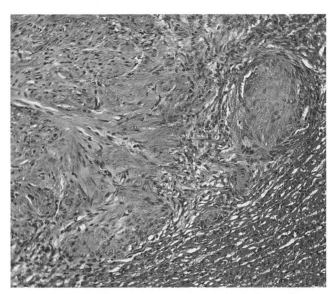

Fig. 1-76 Multicentric infantile myofibromatosis involving myocardium.

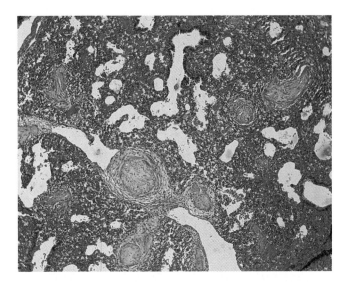

Fig. 1-77 Microscopic appearance of infantile myofibromatosis involving the lungs.

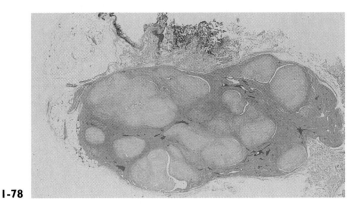

1-78

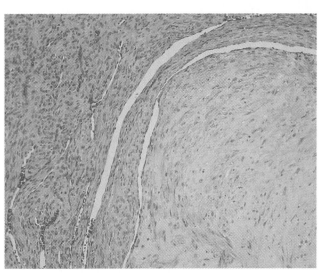

1-79

Figs. 1-78 and 1-79 Some lesions seen in adults are morphologically similar to the solitary myofibromas seen in children, but others demonstrate a broader histologic spectrum with features suggesting a vascular origin and raising the possibility that adult and childhood lesions may not represent the same entity.

Fibromatosis Colli

This fibrous growth occurs in the distal portion of the sternocleidomastoid muscle. Whether it is neoplastic or reparative is unclear; approximately 50% of cases are associated with a history of breech or forceps delivery. However, the lesion may be the cause rather than the result of delivery problems. Localized ischemia occurring during labor could also play a role in its development. It typically presents in the second, third, and fourth weeks of life; affects males more often than females; and involves the right side more often than the left. It is characterized by a growth phase that eventually stabilizes and then regresses. Torticollis or wryneck may develop in either the initial or late stages of the disease.

MICROSCOPIC FEATURES

- Diffuse fibroblastic proliferation within skeletal muscle and subjacent to muscle fascia
- Atrophy of involved musculature
- Absence of inflammatory component
- Hemosiderin deposition (rare)

DIFFERENTIAL DIAGNOSIS

- Fibrodysplasia ossificans progressiva (myositis ossificans progressiva)
- Fibrosing myositis
- Fibromatosis

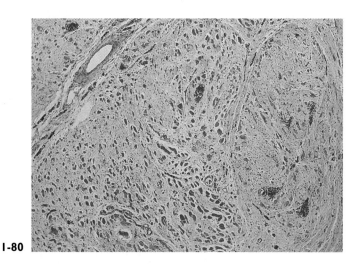
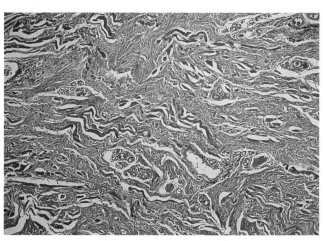

1-80

1-81

Figs. 1-80 and 1-81 Microscopic examples of fibromatosis colli. Note diffuse fibrosis and residual muscle fibers (trichrome stain, Fig. 1-81).

Infantile Digital Fibromatosis

This fibrous proliferation occurs predominantly in the dermis and subcutis of the fingers and toes of infants less than 1 year of age. Approximately 30% of cases are congenital, although rare cases in older children and adults may occur. It is characterized by eosinophilic, globular inclusions that have been shown to be actin by a variety of techniques. Approximately 60% of lesions recur, although most will eventually regress spontaneously. They are capable of causing contracture deformities.

MICROSCOPIC FEATURES

- Fibroblastic fascicles of varying sizes
- Uniform fibroblasts
- Eosinophilic, globular cytoplasmic inclusions (3 to 15 nm)

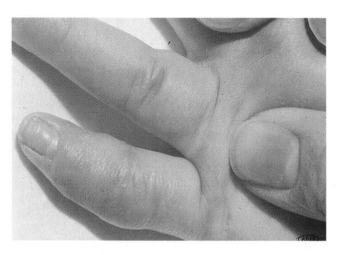

Fig. 1-82 Clinical photograph of infantile digital fibromatosis involving the left fifth digit.

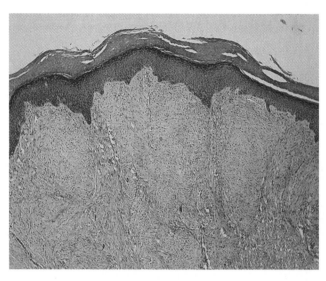

Fig. 1-83 Low magnification of infantile digital fibromatosis demonstrating nodular configuration of lesion.

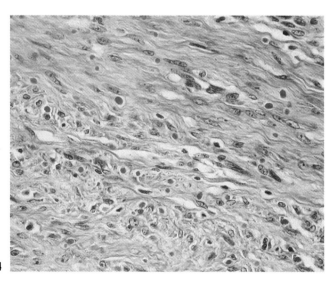

1-84

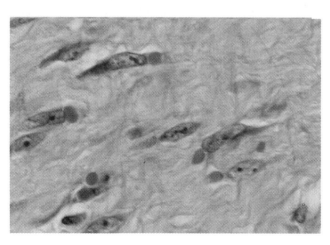

1-85

Figs. 1-84 and 1-85 Eosinophilic globular intracytoplasmic inclusions are a characteristic feature of the fibroblasts in infantile digital fibromatosis.

Infantile Fibromatosis

Infantile fibromatosis is the childhood equivalent of adult-type desmoid or musculoaponeurotic fibromatosis. Generally it is a deep, poorly defined, solitary mass within the skeletal muscle or fascia of children between birth and 5 years of age. The head and neck are the most common sites, followed by the proximal extremities and the limb girdles. The histologic appearance ranges from primitive myxoid mesenchymal lesions (immature diffuse form), which are more common in infants, to those resembling adult desmoids (mature, adult-like form), which are more common in older children. Admixtures of these two types are not uncommon.

Some may recur, be locally aggressive, or involve bone. Neither the location nor the histologic appearance is a useful prognostic feature.

MICROSCOPIC FEATURES

- *Immature, diffuse form*
- Small fibroblast-like cells
- Haphazard arrangement
- Rich reticulin network
- Myxoid matrix
- Diffuse infiltration of muscle
- Atrophic skeletal muscle
- Fatty replacement of muscle
- Lymphoid aggregates

- *Mature, adult-like form*
- Short bundles and fascicles of fibroblasts
- Variable amount of collagen
- Thin-walled ectatic vascular channels
- Scar-like appearance
- Ossification (rare)

DIFFERENTIAL DIAGNOSIS

- Fibrodysplasia ossificans progressiva
- Infantile fibrosarcoma
- Lipoblastomatosis

- Myxoid liposarcoma
- Embryonal rhabdomyosarcoma

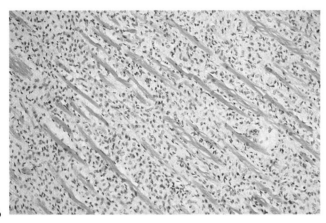

1-86

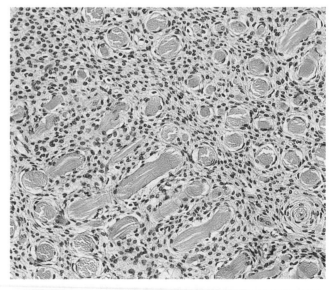

1-87

Figs. 1-86 through 1-89 Immature, diffuse forms of infantile fibromatosis with primitive fibroblasts in a variably fibrous to myxoid matrix infiltrating skeletal muscle. The adjacent adipose tissue may be infiltrated or represent a response to muscle atrophy. Some cases may bear a close resemblance to calcifying aponeurotic fibromas that have not yet calcified.

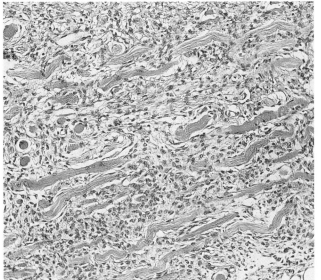

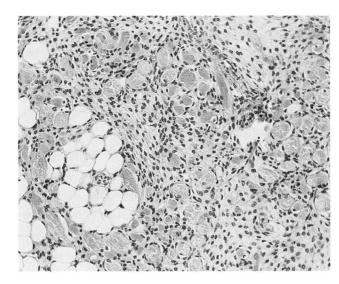

1-88

1-89

Figs. 1-86 through 1-89—cont'd. For legend, see opposite page.

Gingival Fibromatosis

Although gingival fibromatosis is transmitted as an autosomal dominant trait, sporadic cases may occur. It typically presents as a slowly enlarging mass of the upper and lower gingiva and hard palate, usually at the time of eruption of either decidual or permanent teeth. Occasional cases are associated with cherubism, hypertrichosis, mental retardation, and epilepsy.

MICROSCOPIC FEATURES

- Paucicellular
- Dense collagenization
- Acanthosis (variable)

DIFFERENTIAL DIAGNOSIS

- Dilantin hypertrophy
- Chronic gingivitis
- Juvenile hyalin fibromatosis

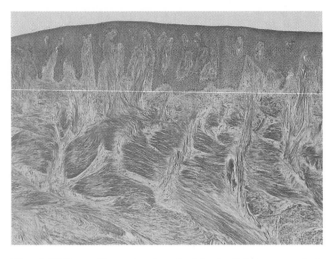

Figs. 1-90 Dense fibrous bands and minimal cellularity are typically seen in gingival fibromatosis.

Calcifying Aponeurotic Fibroma

This slowly growing fibroblastic proliferation occurs primarily in the hands, and to a lesser extent, the feet of children and adolescents; adults are rarely affected. It is a poorly defined, painless mass involving the aponeuroses or tendons. Approximately 50% of cases recur.

MICROSCOPIC FEATURES

- Infiltrative growth pattern
- Central bar-shaped or serpiginous foci of calcification with chondroid areas (variable; absent in early phase)
- Plump, oval fibroblasts
- Dense cellularity (hypercellular)
- Cord-like arrangement of fibroblasts
- Dense, hyalinized collagen
- Giant cells associated with calcification (variable)

DIFFERENTIAL DIAGNOSIS

- Infantile fibromatosis
- Calcifying and non-calcifying chondroma of soft parts
- Tumoral calcinosis
- Palmar or plantar fibromatosis

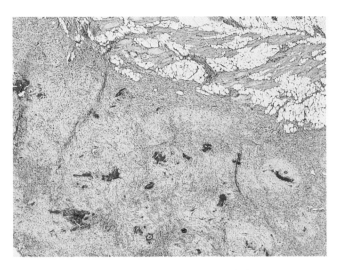

Figs. 1-91 Low magnification appearance of calcifying aponeurotic fibroma demonstrating fibroblastic infiltration of adipose tissue and muscle and discrete areas of calcification.

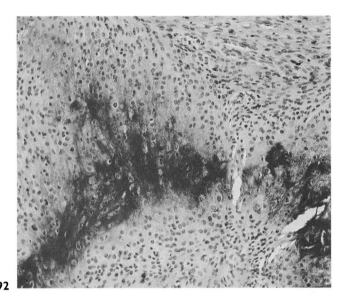

1-92

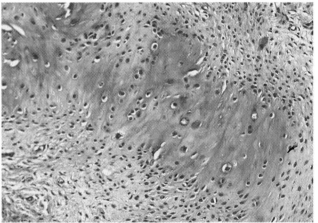

1-93

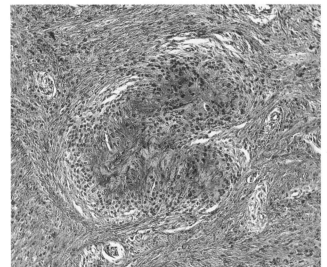

1-94

Figs. 1-92 through 1-94 Bar-shaped and serpiginous zones of calcification are characteristic of calcifying aponeurotic fibroma (trichrome stain, Fig. 1-94).

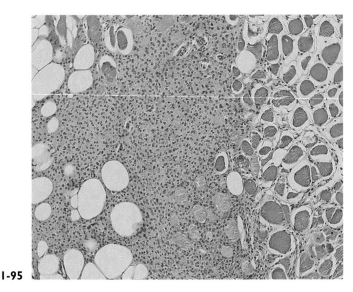

1-95

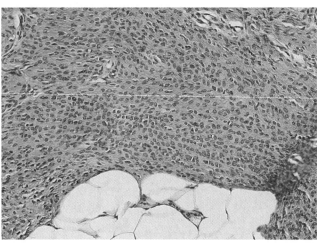

1-96

Figs. 1-95 and 1-96 Proliferation of plump, oval fibroblasts in calcifying aponeurotic fibroma with a cord-like arrangement in some cases (Fig. 1-96). The degree of cellularity is highly variable and may simulate fibrosarcoma.

Juvenile Hyalin Fibromatosis

This rare autosomal recessive disorder is related to faulty collagen metabolism and possibly abnormal synthesis of glycosaminoglycans. Several siblings may be affected. The disease first manifests itself between the ages of 2 and 5 years, usually as mutiple, painless, slowly growing cutaneous nodules on the scalp, ears, nose, knees, and back. Patients may also have thickened gums, flexion contractures, and muscular weakness, as well as multiple osteolytic bone lesions.

MICROSCOPIC FEATURES

- Ill-defined margins
- Small, scattered fibroblast-like cells
- Abundant, amorphous, extracellular, eosinophilic material
- Reticulin and collagen-poor matrix
- Calcification (variable)

DIFFERENTIAL DIAGNOSIS

- Neurofibromatosis
- Gingival fibromatosis
- Lipoid proteinosis
- Winchester's syndrome
- Proteus syndrome

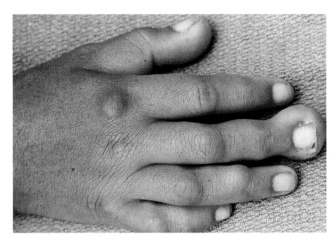

Fig. 1-97 Clinical presentation of hyalin fibromatosis (same case).

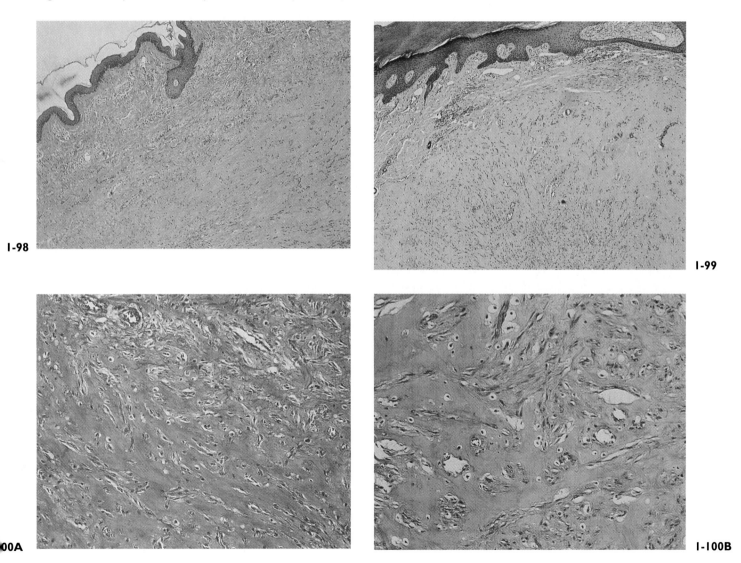

1-98

1-99

00A

1-100B

Figs. 1-98 through 1-100 A paucicellular lesion dominated by an amorphous, eosinophilic matrix with scattered fibroblasts is characteristically seen in hyalin fibromatosis. There is a variable degree of cellularity, and fibroblasts may occasionally cluster around vessels.

Calcifying Fibrous Pseudotumor (with Psammomatous Calcifications)

This fibrous pseudotumor clinically and radiologically mimics a desmoid tumor. Although it was originally described in children, occurrence in young adults has also been documented. It is generally a slowly growing, deep-seated mass that rarely recurs. Associated skeletal or soft tissue lesions have not been described. The etiology is uncertain, although it may represent the end stage of one or a variety of lesions.

MICROSCOPIC FEATURES

- Well-demarcated margins
- Hyalinized, collagenous matrix
- Acellular to hypocellular
- Scattered fibroblasts
- Scattered plasma cells
- Concentric (psammomatous) and dystrophic calcifications
- Russell bodies (variable)
- Rare xanthoma cells and hemosiderin

DIFFERENTIAL DIAGNOSIS

- Amyloidoma
- Myofibroblastic pseudotumor
- Fibroma of tendon sheath

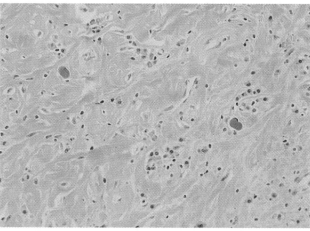
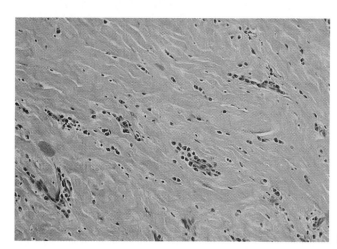

1-101

1-102

Figs. 1-101 and 1-102 Hyalinized zones of collagen contain scattered aggregates of plasma cells. Psammomatous calcifications are usually but not invariably present.

FIBROMATOSES

The fibromatoses are divided into superficial and deep types based on their distinctive morphologic and clinical features.

Superficial Fibromatoses

This group of fibromatoses includes **palmar, plantar,** and **penile fibromatoses,** as well as **knuckle pads.** They are small, slow growing, benign (myo)fibroblastic proliferations that characteristically occur in adults and involve the superficial fascia or aponeuroses. The palmar and plantar aspects of the hands and feet are usually involved. Occasionally they may cause flexion contractures and less often hyperextension. As many as 50% of cases are bilateral, and some may have a hereditary component, as well as an association with epilepsy, diabetes, cirrhosis, or alcoholism.

MICROSCOPIC FEATURES

- Growth along fascia, aponeuroses, and tendons
- Uniform fibroblasts
- Variable cellularity
- Plump to elongated (myo)fibroblasts
- Variable amount of collagenization
- Mitoses (variable)
- Myxoid matrix (variable)
- Cartilaginous or osseous metaplasia (rare)

DIFFERENTIAL DIAGNOSIS

- Cicatrix (scar)
- Infantile fibromatosis
- Calcifying aponeurotic fibroma (early stage)
- Fibrosarcoma

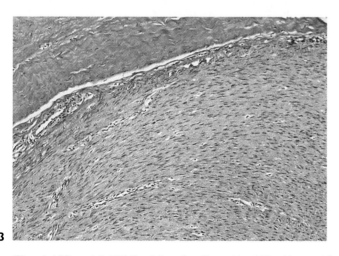
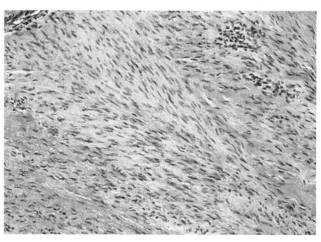

1-103   1-104

Figs. 1-103 and 1-104 Fascicles of uniform, bland fibroblasts with a variable amount of collagen deposition and an intimate association with tendons are typical of palmar fibromatosis, as well as the other superficial fibromatoses.

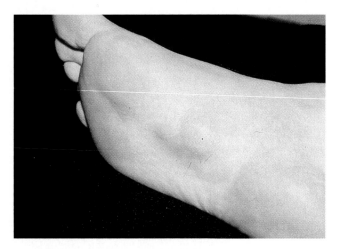

Fig. 1-105 Clinical example of plantar fibromatosis.

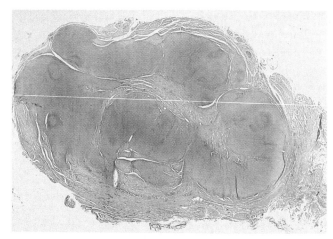

Fig. 1-106 Low magnification of plantar fibromatosis showing intimate association with tendon. The lesions are, in general, relatively well circumscribed.

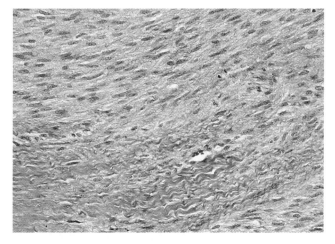

Fig. 1-107 Short fascicles of bland fibroblasts with varying degrees of cellularity and collagen production are seen in plantar fibromatosis.

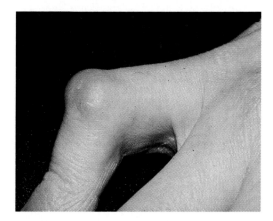

Fig. 1-108 Clinical example of knuckle pad.

Deep Fibromatoses

Deep fibromatoses are most frequently referred to as musculoaponeurotic fibromatosis or desmoid. Like the superficial fibromatoses, there are a variety of distinctive subtypes, including **extra-abdominal fibromatosis** (desmoid), **abdominal fibromatosis** (desmoid), **pelvic fibromatosis, mesenteric fibromatosis,** and **Gardner's syndrome** (familial polyposis associated with mesenteric fibromatosis). The deep fibromatoses occur primarily in adults and typically occur within the deep musculature, its fascia, or aponeuroses with occasional extension into the neighboring subcutis and rarely bone. The shoulder region is the most frequent location, followed by the chest wall, thigh, and mesentery. Occasional cases are multicentric. Abdominal desmoids occur almost exclusively in women who are pregnant or shortly after delivery. Those that occur in the mesentery are associated with a history of prior abdominal surgery in about 50% of cases. Recurrence rates for desmoids, as a whole, range from 25% to 80%.

MICROSCOPIC FEATURES

- Poorly defined, infiltrative margins
- Fascicles
- Broad storiform pattern (primarily abdominal forms)
- Spindled, uniform fibroblasts
- Mitoses (rare)
- Abundant collagen
- Myxoid matrix (primarily abdominal forms)

- Keloid-like collagen foci (rare)
- Rich reticulin network
- Thin-walled, elongated, compressed vessels
- Focal hemorrhage (variable)
- Lymphoid aggregates
- Chondroosseous metaplasia or calcification (rare)

DIFFERENTIAL DIAGNOSIS

- Reactive fibrosis
- Scar (cicatrix)
- Nodular fasciitis

- Myxoma
- Fibrosarcoma

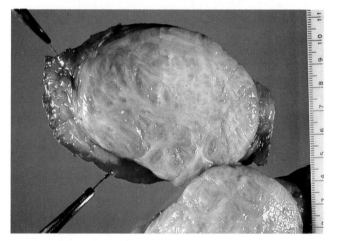

Fig. 1-109 Cut surface of extraabdominal desmoid from the chest wall; the appearance ranges from tan and fleshy to white and fibrous, depending on the amount of myxoid matrix and collagen. The apparent circumscription is deceptive; most of these lesions infiltrate along fascial planes.

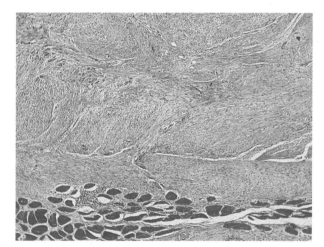

1-110

Figs. 1-110 through 1-116 Typical examples of musculoaponeurotic fibromatosis showing fascicular arrangements of bland fibroblasts, which are interrupted by thin-walled, compressed vascular channels resulting in an appearance akin to a hypercellular scar. Note entrapped muscle fibers (Figs. 1-110 and 1-114; trichrome stains, Figs. 1-110 and 1-116).

(Figs continued on next page.)

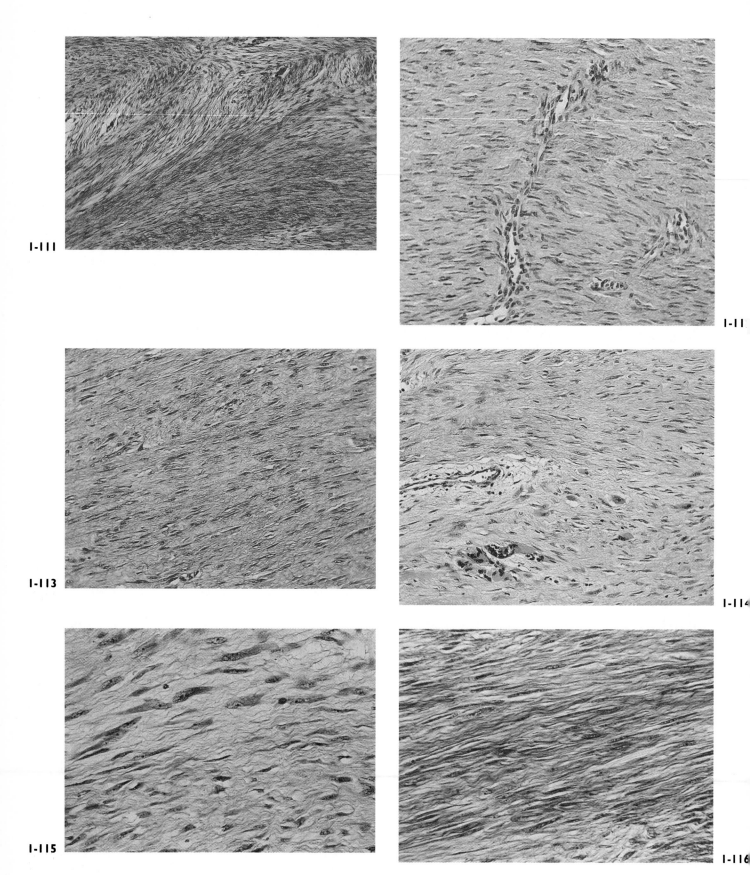

1-111

1-11

1-113

1-114

1-115

1-116

Figs. 1-110 through 1-116—cont'd. For legend, see page 37.

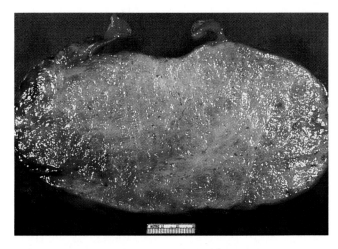

Fig. 1-117 Gross example of mesenteric fibromatosis.

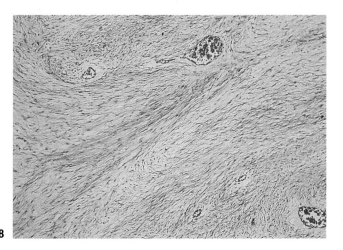

1-118

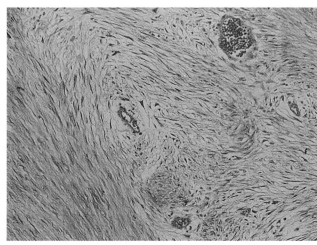

1-119

Figs. 1-118 and 1-119 Mesenteric fibromatoses (mesenteric desmoids) are frequently more myxoid than those seen within the deep musculature or retroperitoneum. One of these (Fig. 1-117) arose in the mesentery of a patient with Gardner's syndrome.

MALIGNANT

Adult Fibrosarcoma

Adult fibrosarcoma is a deep-seated, slow-growing, and usually painless mass occurring primarily in patients in the fourth through sixth decades of life. It most frequently occurs in the lower extremities, followed by the upper extremities, trunk, and the head and neck region. Intramuscular fibrous tissue, aponeuroses, and tendons are frequently involved by fibrosarcoma, as are adjacent nerves and vessels. Involvement of the subcutis is rare unless there is association with dermatofibrosarcoma protuberans, a prior scar (cicatricial), burn, or history of radiation therapy (radiation-induced fibrosarcoma). Fibrosarcoma is in general a diagnosis of exclusion.

MICROSCOPIC FEATURES

- Fascicles and herringbone architecture
- Uniform fibroblasts with scant cytoplasm
- Small round to oval cells (rare)
- Mitoses, occasionally atypical
- Dense network of collagen fibrils and variable fibrosis

- Fibroma or fibromatosis-like areas (variable)
- Myxoid matrix (variable)
- Necrosis (variable)
- Osseous or chondroid metaplasia (rare)

DIFFERENTIAL DIAGNOSIS

- Nodular fasciitis
- Fibrous histiocytoma
- Fibromatosis
- Monophasic synovial sarcoma, fibrous type

- Malignant fibrous histiocytoma
- Malignant peripheral nerve sheath tumor (malignant schwannoma, neurofibrosarcoma)
- Sarcomatoid carcinoma

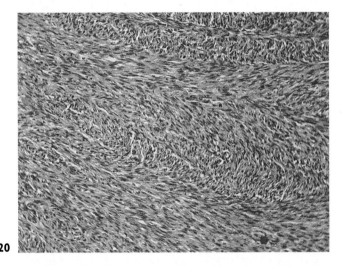

1-120

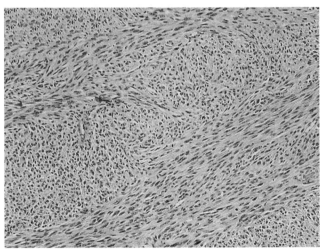

1-121

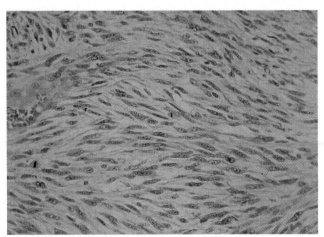

1-122

Figs. 1-120 through 1-124 Intertwining fascicles of relatively uniform fibroblasts and a variable amount of collagen deposition are seen in adult fibrosarcoma. The fascicles are usually arranged at acute angles to each other, resulting in a herringbone appearance. Occasionally the cells may assume a more rounded appearance, and there may be abundant extracellular deposition of collagen-simulating osteoid. In other instances, there may be a prominent myxoid stroma.

(Figs continued on next page.)

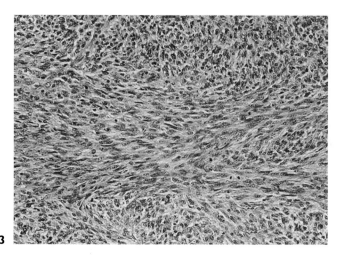

1-123

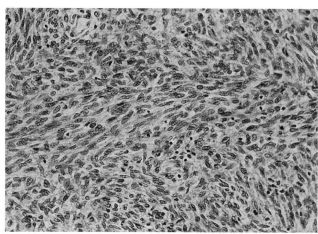

1-124

Figs. 1-120 through 1-124—cont'd. For legend, see opposite page.

Congenital and Infantile Fibrosarcoma

This neoplasm occurs primarily in children 1 year of age or less; about 20% are congenital. It typically presents as a large, painless mass with a predilection for the distal extremities. Cortical ero-sion of underlying bone, bowing, and occasional bone destruction may also occur. Infantile fibrosarcoma tends to have a much better prognosis than its adult counterpart despite ominous histologic features such as necrosis and hemorrhage.

MICROSCOPIC FEATURES

- Fascicular architecture (sometimes illdefined)
- Spindled to round, small, primitive fibroblasts
- Dense network of collagen fibrils
- Lymphocytic infiltrate
- Frequent mitoses
- Necrosis
- Hemorrhage

DIFFERENTIAL DIAGNOSIS

- Fibrous hamartoma of infancy
- Myofibromatosis
- Fibromatosis
- Embryonal rhabdomyosarcoma
- Infantile hemangiopericytoma
- Spindle cell angiosarcoma

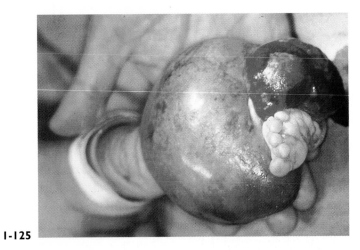

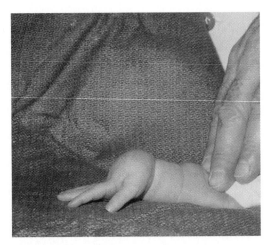

1-125

1-126

Figs. 1-125 and 1-126 Clinical photographs of infantile fibrosarcoma involving the foot (Fig. 1-125) and hand (Fig. 1-126).

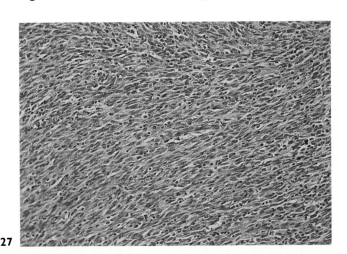

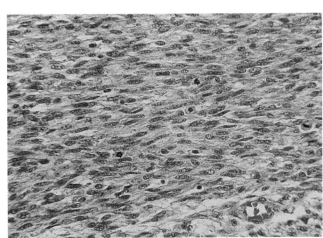

1-127

1-128

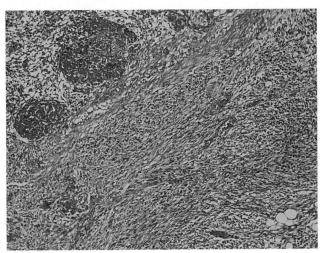

1-129

Figs. 1-127 through 1-129 Closely packed spindled fibroblasts arrange in ill-defined fascicles are seen in infantile fibrosarcoma. Round to angulated primitive fibroblasts associated with a lymphocytic infiltrate may also be seen. Mitotic figures are readily identified. Focal vascularization may simulate an angiosarcoma (Fig. 1-129).

Inflammatory Fibrosarcoma

Inflammatory fibrosarcoma occurs primarily but not exclusively in infants and young children. It typically presents as multiple nodules or masses within the abdominal cavity, retroperitoneum, and mesentery and is associated with systemic symptoms such as fever, anemia, weight loss, and elevated erythrocyte sedimentation rate. Unlike myofibroblastic pseudotumors in other sites, inflammatory fibrosarcoma does not regress spontaneously. Although some patients are cured by local excision, others experience local recurrences and rarely metastases.

MICROSCOPIC FEATURES

- Fascicular architecture
- Fibroblasts and myofibroblasts
- Ganglion cell–like myofibroblasts
- Collagen deposition (fibrils or hyalinized)
- Inflammation (usually plasma cells)
- Calcification (variable)
- Myxoid matrix (variable)

DIFFERENTIAL DIAGNOSIS

- Inflammatory myofibroblastic pseudotumor
- Leiomyosarcoma
- Malignant fibrous histiocytoma

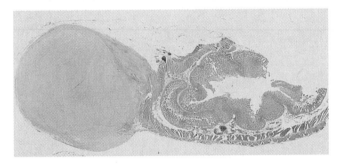

Fig. I-130 Whole-mount section of an inflammatory fibrosarcoma involving the small intestine (trichrome stain).

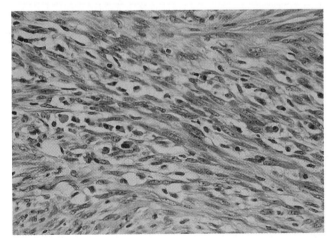

Fig. I-131 Elongated atypical (myo)fibroblastic cells are arranged in fascicles and are associated with an inflammatory infiltrate that usually consists of lymphocytes and plasma cells. Although the cells of inflammatory fibrosarcoma may closely resemble smooth muscle, cytoplasmic basophilia and sharply tapered or pointed nuclei are indicative of (myo)fibroblastic differentiation.

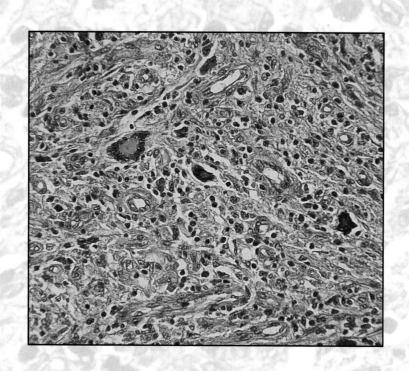

Chapter 2

Fibrohistiocytic Tumors

BENIGN

Fibrous Histiocytoma

Fibrous histiocytoma is a slow-growing, painless, benign lesion that occurs in the dermis and subcutis. It is composed of fibroblasts, myofibroblasts, and histiocytes, often arranged in a storiform pattern. Intramuscular and visceral lesions are rare. Most fibrous histiocytomas occur on the extremities, primarily during the third through fifth decades of life. Multiple metachronous lesions are more common in cutaneous than deep fibrous histiocytomas. Recurrence rates range between 5% and 10%. The superficial or cutaneous lesions tend to be smaller and have a more heterogeneous cell population with a variety of inflammatory cells and secondary changes, such as siderophages and hemorrhage, than the more deeply situated subcutaneous lesions, which are predominantly (myo)-fibroblastic.

MICROSCOPIC FEATURES

- Well-defined to focally infiltrative margins
- Storiform pattern
- Short fascicles
- Hemangiopericytoma pattern (rare)
- Spindled to oval fibroblasts
- Round to oval histiocytoid cells
- Multinucleated, osteoclast-like, or Touton giant cells
- Myxoid change
- Collagen deposition
- Hyalinization
- Hemorrhage, hemosiderin
- Xanthoma cells
- Inflammatory cells

DIFFERENTIAL DIAGNOSIS

- Nodular fasciitis
- Neurofibroma
- Leiomyoma
- Hemangiopericytoma
- Reaction to foreign materials (e.g., silica, polyvinylpyrrolidone)
- Infectious agents (e.g., leprosy)
- Rosai-Dorfman disease of soft tissue
- Histiocytic "granular" cell reaction
- Dermatofibrosarcoma protuberans
- Malignant fibrous histiocytoma (MFH)
- Angiomatoid MFH
- Kaposi's sarcoma

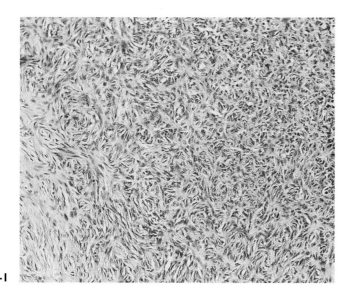

2-1

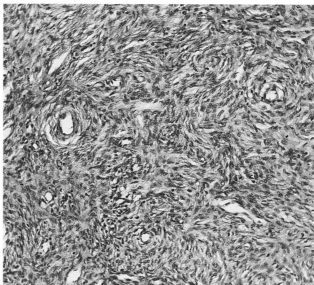

2-2

Figs. 2-1 through 2-3 Typical examples of fibrous histiocytoma exhibiting a distinct storiform pattern. The cell population in these examples is relatively homogeneous and consists of "fibrohistiocytic" cells (fibroblasts with a limited number of histiocytic features).

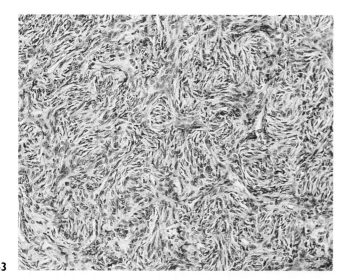

2-3

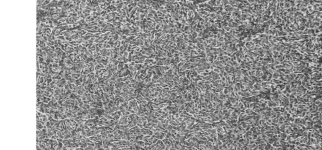

2-4

Figs. 2-4 and 2-5 Examples of cellular fibrous histiocytoma. Epithelioid histiocytes with abundant eosinophilic cytoplasm may be seen focally or may be the predominant component in a fibrous histiocytoma as seen in Fig. 2-5**B**. Epithelioid fibrous histiocytomas may be confused with a Spitz nevus or a reticulohistiocytoma.

(Figs continued on next page.)

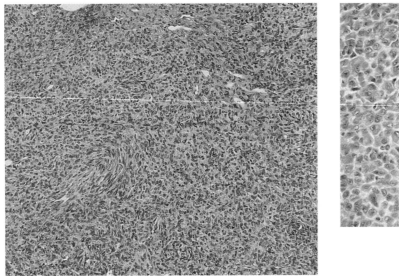

2-5A

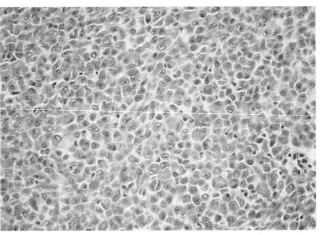

2-5B

Figs. 2-4 and 2-5—cont'd. For legend, see page 47.

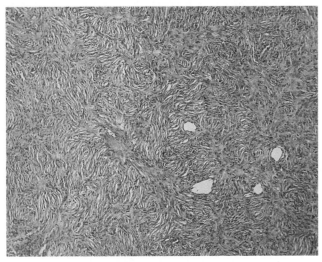

2-6

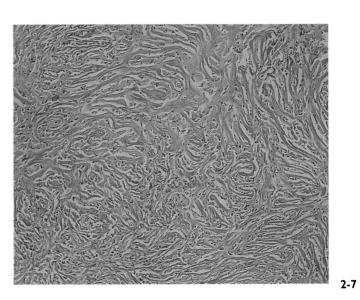

2-7

Figs. 2-6 and 2-7 A variable degree of sclerosis may be seen in fibrous histiocytoma. Sometimes it is so extensive that the underlying lesion is nearly obscured, but the storiform pattern remains.

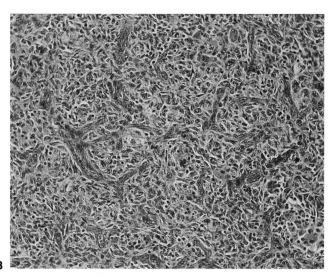

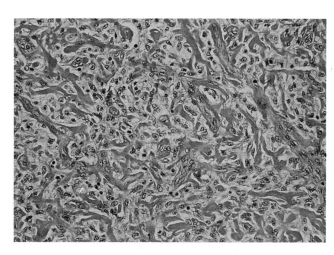

2-8

2-9

Figs. 2-8 and 2-9 Fibrous histiocytomas with a prominent vasculature. Some fibrous histiocytomas may have prominent sclerosis of the blood vessel walls. When the vascular pattern is hemangiopericytic, distinction from hemangiopericytoma may be difficult.

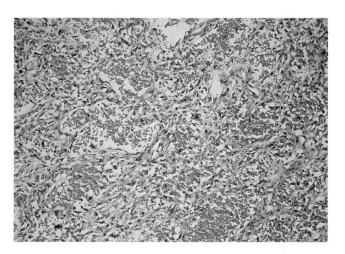

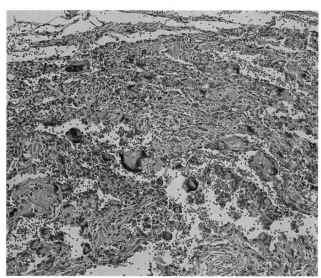

Fig. 2-10 Cellular fibrous histiocytoma with hemorrhage. These cases could be mistaken for angiomatoid malignant fibrous histiocytoma.

Fig. 2-11 Gaping cystic spaces resulting from loss of cellular cohesion and hemorrhage create a pseudovascular pattern in this fibrous histiocytoma with scattered bizarre giant cells.

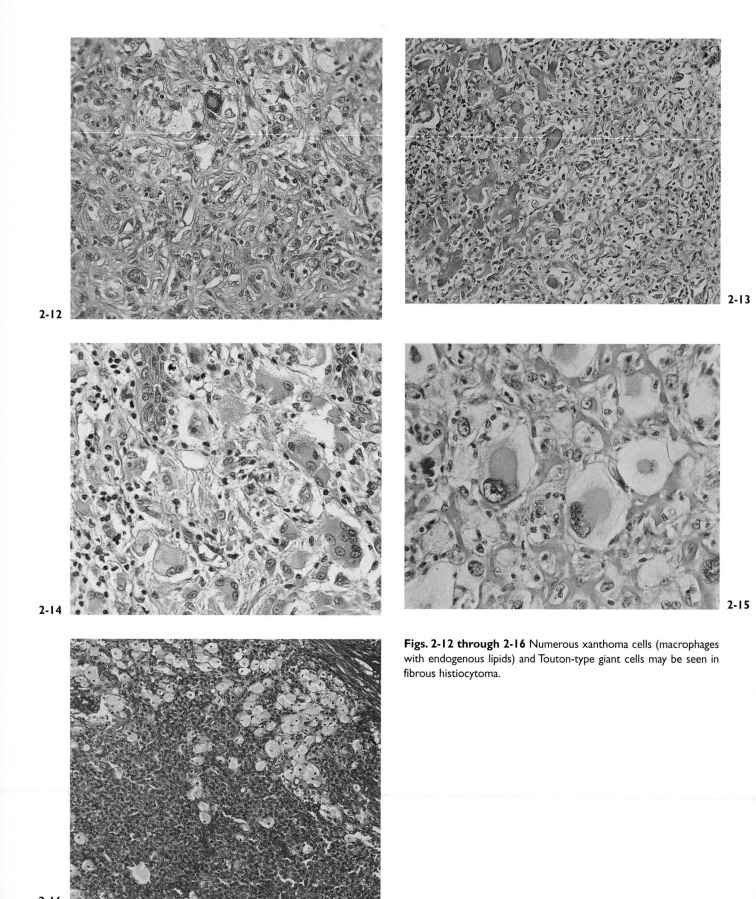

Figs. 2-12 through 2-16 Numerous xanthoma cells (macrophages with endogenous lipids) and Touton-type giant cells may be seen in fibrous histiocytoma.

Juvenile Xanthogranuloma

This fibrohistiocytic proliferation of infancy typically occurs within the first 6 months of life (20% are congenital) and rarely in adults (10%). The cutaneous form of this disease is most common, with one to multiple red nodules gradually regressing to a tan macule or depression on the skin surface. Less commonly (about 5%) deep soft tissue sites or other organs such as the eye are involved. Despite the presence of intracytoplasmic lipid, there is no associated lipid abnormality. Whether juvenile xanthogranuloma is a reactive or neoplastic proliferation of benign histiocytes is uncertain, but the self-limited, regressive course in most cases suggests a reactive process.

MICROSCOPIC FEATURES

- Well-defined to infiltrative margins
- Uniform histiocytes
- Eosinophilic to vacuolated to xanthomatous cytoplasm
- Touton giant cells (variable)
- Eosinophils
- Other acute and chronic inflammatory cells
- Sclerosis (with regression)

DIFFERENTIAL DIAGNOSIS

- Histiocytosis X
- Fibrous histiocytoma
- Xanthoma

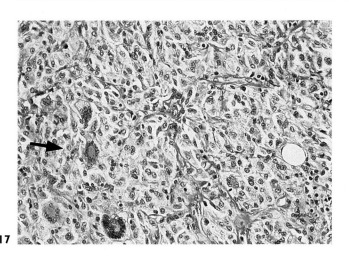

2-17

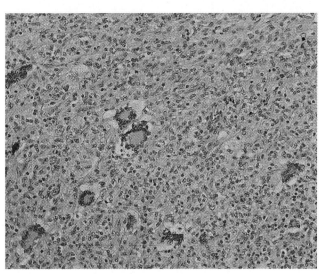

2-18

Figs. 2-17 and 2-18 Typical cases of juvenile xanthogranuloma with scattered Touton giant cells (*arrow*) amid a background of mononuclear eosinophilic to vacuolated histiocytes.

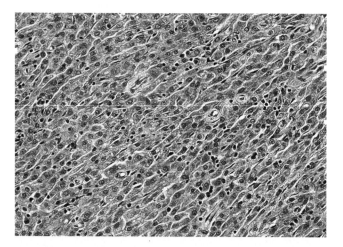

Fig. 2-19 A juvenile xanthogranuloma with epithelioid histiocytes and absence of Touton giant cells.

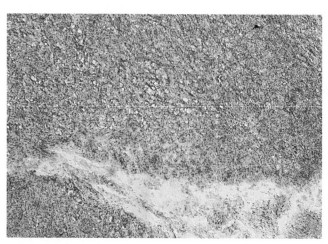

Fig. 2-20 The oil red O stain demonstrates the presence of neutral lipids in the mononuclear cells of juvenile xanthogranuloma.

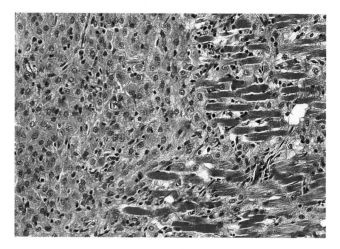

Fig. 2-21 Deep juvenile xanthogranuloma with epithelioid histiocytes infiltrating skeletal muscle.

Reticulohistiocytoma

Reticulohistiocytoma most frequently occurs as a single, red-brown, cutaneous nodule of the upper portion of the body in adults; approximately 20% of cases are associated with multiple skin lesions. It is characterized by a proliferation of relatively uniform histiocytes with abundant, glassy, eosinophilic cytoplasm within the dermis. A rare, systemic form of the disease, which may involve the synovium, lymph nodes, bone, and heart, is sometimes associated with debilitating arthritis, multiple mucocutaneous nodules, fever, and weight loss, and tends to have an undulating course. Whether this is a reactive or neoplastic process is unknown.

MICROSCOPIC FEATURES

- Circumscription
- Relatively uniform histiocytes
- Abundant, eosinophilic, "glassy" cytoplasm
- Multinucleated histiocytes
- Spindled histiocytes or fibroblasts (variable)
- Inflammation

DIFFERENTIAL DIAGNOSIS

■ Malignant fibrous histiocytoma   ■ Melanoma

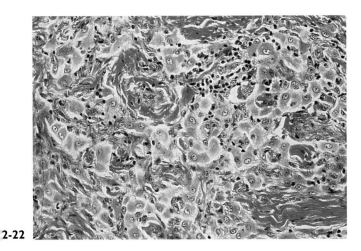

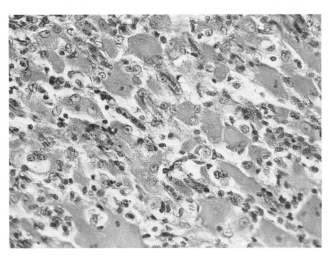

2-22   2-23

Figs. 2-22 and 2-23 Epithelioid histiocytes with abundant, glassy eosinophilic cytoplasm and scattered inflammatory cells characterize the reticulohistiocytoma.

Xanthoma

Xanthomas are reactive proliferations of histiocytes that usually contain abundant intracytoplasmic lipid and are frequently, but not exclusively, associated with hyperlipidemia. They usually occur in the skin and subcutis; less commonly they involve tendons or synovium. The various types of xanthomas are largely related to the type of lipid disorder and anatomic location: eruptive, tuberous, tendinous, plane xanthomas, and xanthelasmas.

MICROSCOPIC FEATURES

■ Circumscribed or diffuse lesions
■ Sheets of histiocytes
■ Foamy and nonfoamy histiocytes
■ Fibrosis (variable)

■ Cholesterol crystals (clefts) surrounded by multinucleated giant cells
■ Hemosiderin

DIFFERENTIAL DIAGNOSIS

■ Giant cell tumor of tendon sheath
■ Pigmented villonodular synovitis

■ Lipogranuloma
■ Malignant fibrous histiocytoma

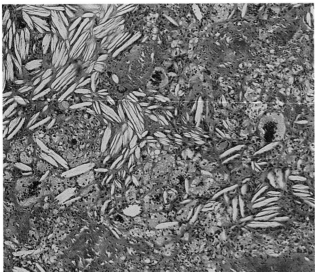
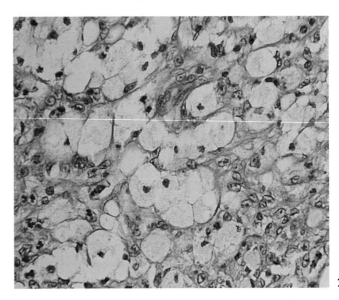

Figs. 2-24 and 2-25 Foamy lipid-laden macrophages, cholesterol clefts, and multinucleated giant cells are seen in varying proportions in the various types of xanthoma.

LOW-GRADE MALIGNANT

Dermatofibrosarcoma Protuberans

Dermatofibrosarcoma protuberans (DFSP) is a low-grade sarcoma that typically involves the dermis and subcutis of young adults. It generally occurs on the trunk or the extremities. In its initial phases, DFSP presents as either a plaque or small nodules that grow slowly and eventually progresses to the classic, multinodular, protuberant stage. Local recurrences are common and occur in about 30% to 60% of cases, indicating the need for complete local excision. Metastases are extremely rare (<5% of cases) and most frequently occur in lungs and lymph nodes; they are more frequent in cases with multiple recurrences. Transformation to higher-grade sarcomas such as fibrosarcoma or MFH may occur in a minority of DFSPs, but its prognostic significance at this time is unknown. The histogenesis of DFSP is also uncertain, but most studies suggest it is fibroblastic rather than neural.

MICROSCOPIC FEATURES

- Diffusely infiltrative margins
- Dermal and/or subcutaneous distribution
- Monotonous, uniform, and redundant storiform pattern
- Pinwheel orientation centered around small vessels
- Homogeneous population of spindled, fibroblast-like cells
- Minimal collagen
- Myxoid zones with attenuation of storiform pattern
- Transitions to fibrosarcoma and MFH (occasional)
- Multinucleated giant cells in deeper portion of tumor (rare)

DIFFERENTIAL DIAGNOSIS

- Fibrous histiocytoma
- Diffuse neurofibroma
- Fibrosarcoma
- Myxoid liposarcoma
- MFH

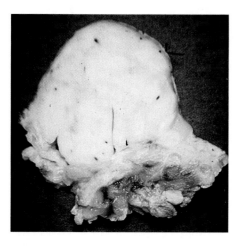

Fig. 2-26 Gross specimen of DFSP demonstrating protuberant growth from the subcutis.

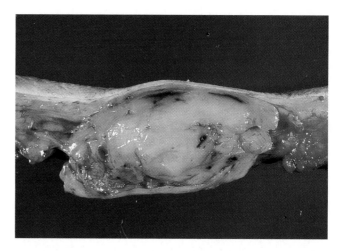

Fig. 2-27 Gross specimen of DFSP showing a predominantly dermal tumor with only slight elevation of the overlying epidermis.

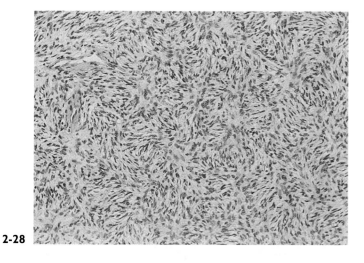

2-28

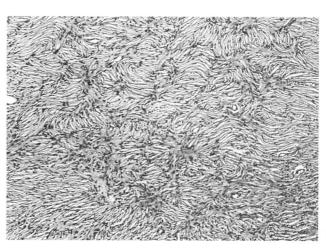

2-29

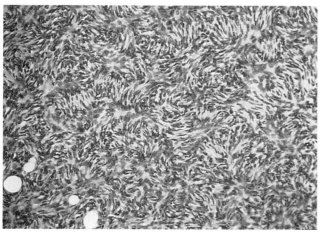

2-30

2-31

Figs. 2-28 through 2-31 A redundant, uniform storiform pattern and relatively bland nuclear features are characteristic of DFSP.

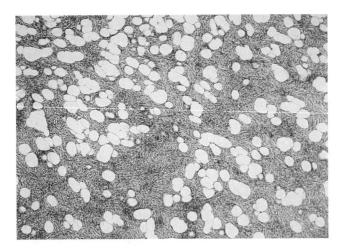

Fig. 2-32 A case of DFSP diffusely infiltrating fat; the storiform pattern is seen better in areas that do not infiltrate fat.

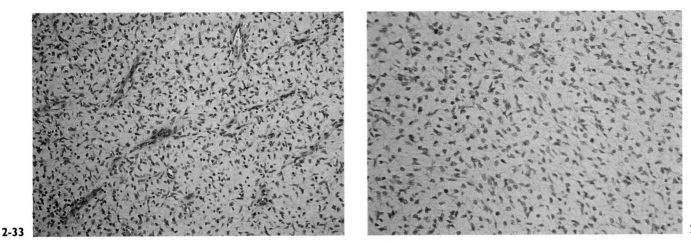

2-33

2-34

Figs. 2-33 and 2-34 The myxoid variant of DFSP may be extremely difficult to diagnosis in the absence of classic areas of DFSP, primarily because the storiform pattern is obscured by an abundant myxoid matrix. However, the superficial location, monotony of the cell proliferation, infiltrative pattern, absence of lipoblasts, and delicate vascularity are important clues in diagnosis.

Giant Cell Fibroblastoma

Giant cell fibroblastoma occurs primarily but not exclusively in children. It is a slow-growing, painless mass that tends to occur on the trunk and primarily involves the dermis and subcutis. Approximately half the cases recur locally. A relationship to DFSP has been postulated on the basis of rare overlapping histologic features.

MICROSCOPIC FEATURES

- Pseudosinusoidal or gaping spaces simulating vascular channels
- Multinucleated giant fibroblast-like cells (frequently around the pseudosinusoidal spaces)
- Elongated fibroblast-like cells
- Fibrous to myxoid matrix
- Occasional storiform foci resembling DFSP

DIFFERENTIAL DIAGNOSIS

- Fibrous histiocytoma
- Myxoma
- Myxoid lipoblastoma
- Myxoid liposarcoma
- Myxoid malignant fibrous histiocytoma

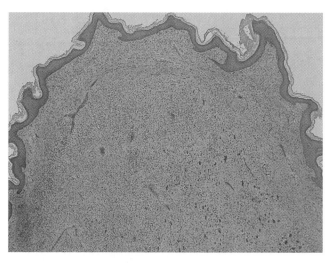

Fig. 2-35 Low magnification of giant cell fibroblastomas (GCF) illustrating the superficial location of the lesion.

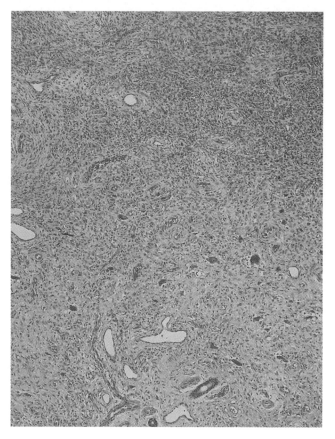

Fig. 2-36 A case of GCF with bland fibroblastic areas reminiscent of DFSP.

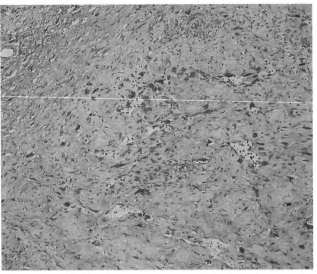

2-37A

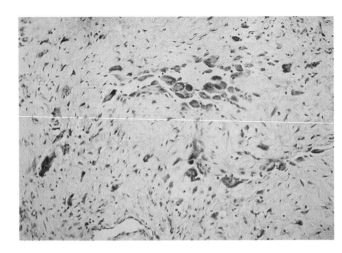

2-37

Fig. 2-37 A, B Pseudosinusoidal gaping spaces associated with large multinucleated fibroblast-like cells characteristic of GCF.

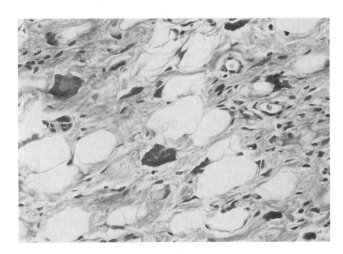

Fig. 2-38 Enlarged fibroblast-like cells with multiple nuclei; the nuclei typically overlap and are hyperchromatic.

Bednar Tumor

Clinically and histologically, this lesion is nearly identical to DFSP with the exception of the presence of a variable amount of melanin pigment with-in melanosomes of lesional cells. The behavior of Bednar tumor is presumed to be similar to that of DFSP, but the number of reported cases is small.

MICROSCOPIC FEATURES

■ See DFSP—Microscopic features

■ Melanin-laden cells with dendritic processes

DIFFERENTIAL DIAGNOSIS

- See DFSP—Differential diagnosis
- Cellular blue nevus
- Melanoma

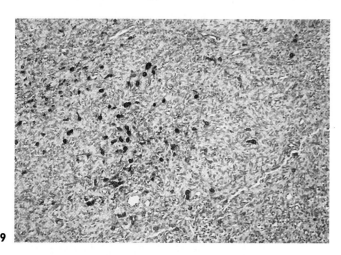

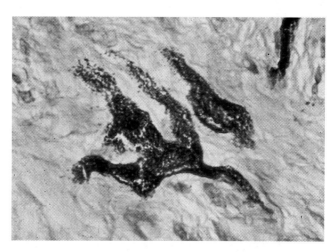

2-39

2-40

Figs. 2-39 and 2-40 Examples of Bednar tumor showing a storiform spindle cell pattern, indistinguishable from that of DFSP, punctuated by melanin-laden dendritic cells.

Plexiform Fibrohistiocytic Tumor

This fibrohistiocytic proliferation tends to occur in children and involves the deep dermis and subcutis of the upper extremities and shoulder region. Roughly one third of cases recur locally; two cases with regional lymph node metastases have been documented; however, no tumor deaths have been reported. In all likelihood, the tumor is a variant of fibrous histiocytoma and somewhat akin to benign, metastasizing fibrous histiocytoma.

MICROSCOPIC FEATURES

- Plexiform to multinodular architecture
- Dermal and subcutaneous distribution
- Oval to spindled fibrohistiocytic cells
- Fibroblasts
- Osteoclast-like multinucleated giant cells
- Collagen between nodules
- Hemosiderin
- Vascular invasion (rare)

DIFFERENTIAL DIAGNOSIS

- Fibromatosis
- Plexiform neurofibroma
- Fibrous histiocytoma
- Myofibroma
- Fibrous hamartoma of infancy
- MFH

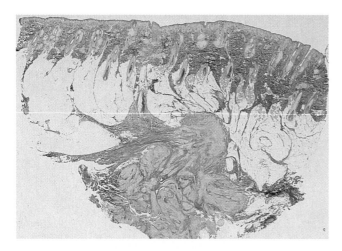

Fig. 2-41 Low magnification of plexiform fibrohistiocytic tumor (PFHT) demonstrating involvement of the deep subcutis and a multinodular to plexiform architecture (trichrome stain).

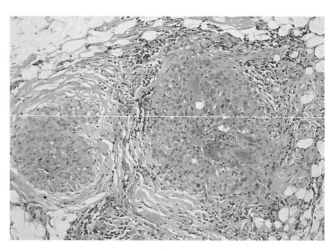

Fig. 2-42 A predominantly fibrohistiocytic cell population with scattered osteoclast-like giant cells is seen in this example of PFHT.

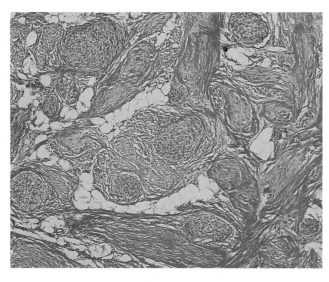

Fig. 2-43 Example of PFHT with a mixture of fibrohistiocytic and fibroblastic cells types.

Fig. 2-44 A, PFHT consisting almost exclusively of a fibroblastic proliferation. These lesions are frequently confused with plexiform neurofibroma, fibromatosis, and fibrous hamartoma of infancy. **B,** PFHT demonstrating vascular invasion; this feature does not portend metastasis.

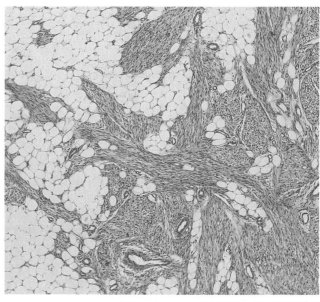

2-44

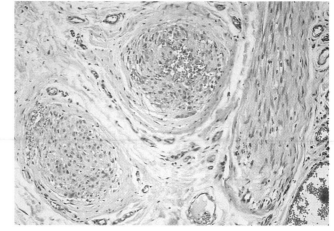

2-44B

Atypical Fibroxanthoma

Atypical fibroxanthoma is a superficial variant of MFH that typically occurs in actinically damaged skin of the head and neck, frequently in elderly individuals. Less often it may involve the trunk and limbs of younger patients. It has an almost uniformly good prognosis because it is a relatively small, superficial lesion in which complete surgical extirpation is usually readily achieved.

MICROSCOPIC FEATURES

- Dermis and upper subcutis
- Fascicular or storiform pattern (variable)
- Haphazardly arranged cells
- Pleomorphic, bizarre cells
- Abundant, eosinophilic cytoplasm, vacuolated to glassy
- Mitoses (typical and atypical)
- Collagenization (variable)
- Myxoid matrix (variable)

DIFFERENTIAL DIAGNOSIS

- Fibrous histioctyoma
- Malignant fibrous histiocytoma
- Melanoma
- Carcinoma
- Leiomyosarcoma

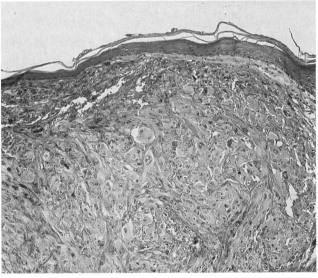
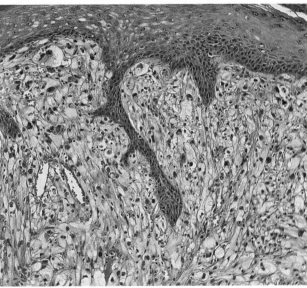

Figs. 2-45 and 2-46 Various examples of atypical fibroxanthoma illustrating the superficial nature and bizarre cell population characteristic of the lesion. They are histologically indistinguishable from MFH. Scattered inflammatory cells are frequently present, and actinic damage is usually observed in the adjacent skin.

Angiomatoid Malignant Fibrous Histiocytoma

Angiomatoid MFH tends to occur in the subcutis and deep dermis of the upper extremities of young patients and is characterized by a propensity for local recurrences if incompletely excised, as well as rare metastases to lungs and lymph nodes.

Clinically, it is a slow-growing mass that is fluctuant and discolored due to hemorrhage. The lesion may be associated with fever, weight loss, and anemia. The prognosis is excellent, provided the lesion has been completely removed. The cell of origin is disputed, although the preponderance of evidence to date supports a fibrohistiocytic origin.

MICROSCOPIC FEATURES

- Well circumscribed
- Fibrous pseudocapsule
- Relatively uniform histiocytoid cell population
- Syncytial to whorled arrangement of cells
- Cystic hemorrhage (central)
- Cuff of lymphocytes and plasma cells (peripheral)
- Hemosiderin
- Focal myxoid change (variable)
- Pleomorphism (rare)

DIFFERENTIAL DIAGNOSIS

- Hemorrhagic fibrous histiocytoma
- MFH
- Myxoid MFH
- Metastatic melanoma (or other metastatic neoplasms)

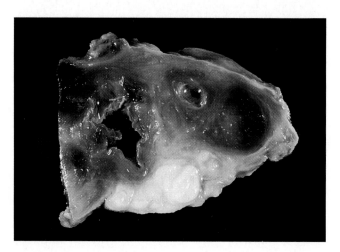

Fig. 2-47 Gross specimen of angiomatoid-MFH demonstrating circumscribed, hemorrhagic, and cystic spaces.

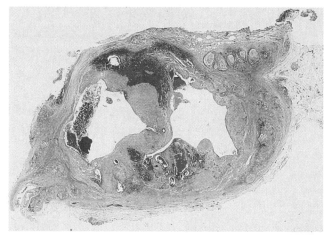

Fig. 2-48 Classic appearance of an angiomatoid malignant fibrous histiocytoma (angiomatoid-MFH); the lesion involves the subcutis and is relatively well circumscribed, hemorrhagic, and cystic.

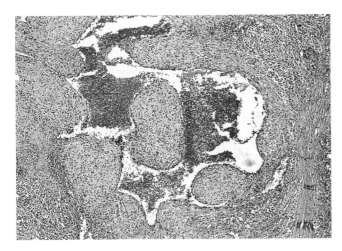

Fig. 2-49 The histiocytoid cells comprising A-MFH are typically arranged in a syncytium wherein the cell boundaries are ill defined. The cystic spaces are typically filled with blood; neither vessel wall nor endothelium is seen lining these areas.

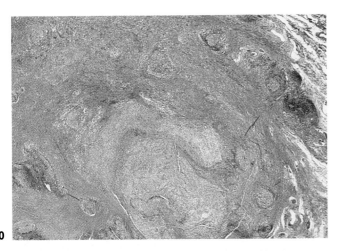

2-50

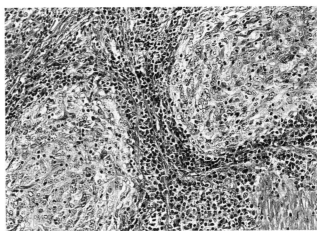

2-51

Figs. 2-50 through 2-52 A cuff of lymphoid tissue, with or without germinal centers, is one of the characteristic features of A-MFH. Neither a lymph node capsule nor sinuses are identified; however, plasma cells and siderophages are characteristically present.

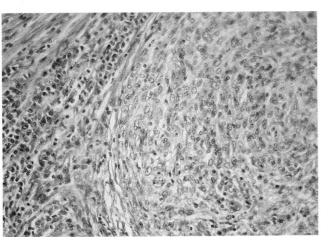

2-52

MALIGNANT

Malignant Fibrous Histiocytoma

MFH is probably the most common sarcoma of adults. It occurs mainly in the sixth and seventh decades of life. Depth and to a lesser extent location are key prognostic factors, as is histologic subtype. All of the subcategories of MFH tend to occur primarily in the extremities, followed by the retroperitoneum; an exception is inflammatory MFH, which occurs primarily in the retroperitoneum. In general the local recurrence rate ranges from 40% to 60%, and the metastatic rate, from 25% to 50%; the myxoid and inflammtory types tend to have lower rates of metastases, and the myxoid type has a higher rate of local recurrence. The propensity to grow in a multinodular fashion and extend into fascial planes probably accounts for the high rate of recurrence in MFH. Metastases to the lungs are most frequent, followed by lymph nodes, liver, and bone. MFH displays primarily fibroblastic and myofibroblastic differentiation in addition to having histiocytoid features; it is largely a diagnosis of exclusion.

Storiform/Pleomorphic MFH

MICROSCOPIC FEATURES

- Storiform or pinwheel pattern
- Short fascicles
- Bizarre, pleomorphic cells
- Uniform fibroblastic cells
- Atypical mitoses
- Xanthoma cells
- Chronic inflammation
- Hyalinization
- Necrosis

DIFFERENTIAL DIAGNOSIS

- Benign fibrous histiocytoma
- DFSP
- Pleomorphic liposarcoma
- Pleomorphic rhabdomyosarcoma
- Poorly differentiated carcinoma

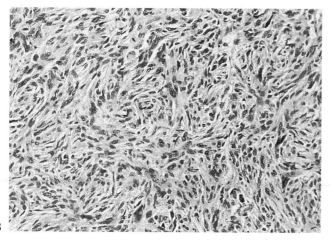

2-53

Figs. 2-53 through 2-56 A storiform pattern, atypical/pleomorphic cells, and scattered inflammatory cells characterize these examples of storiform MFH. Some of these infiltrate adjacent adipose tissue.

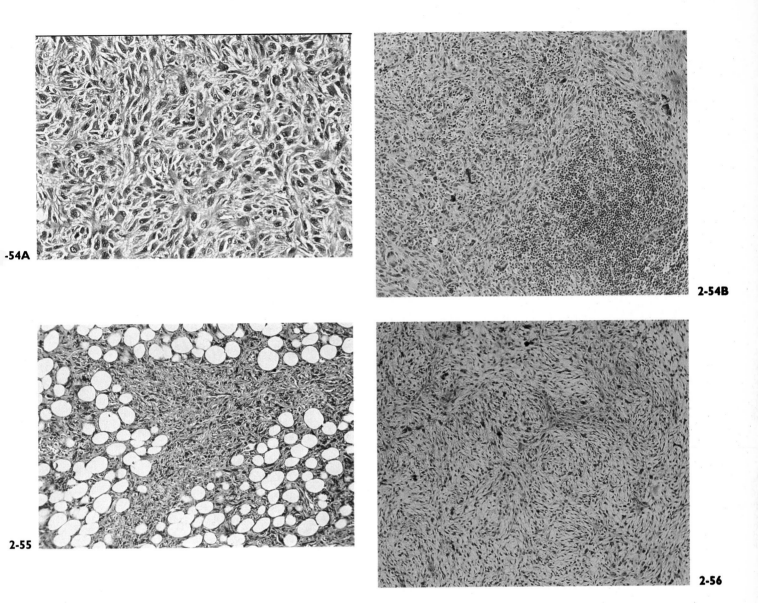

Figs. 2-53 through 2-56—cont'd. For legend, see opposite page.

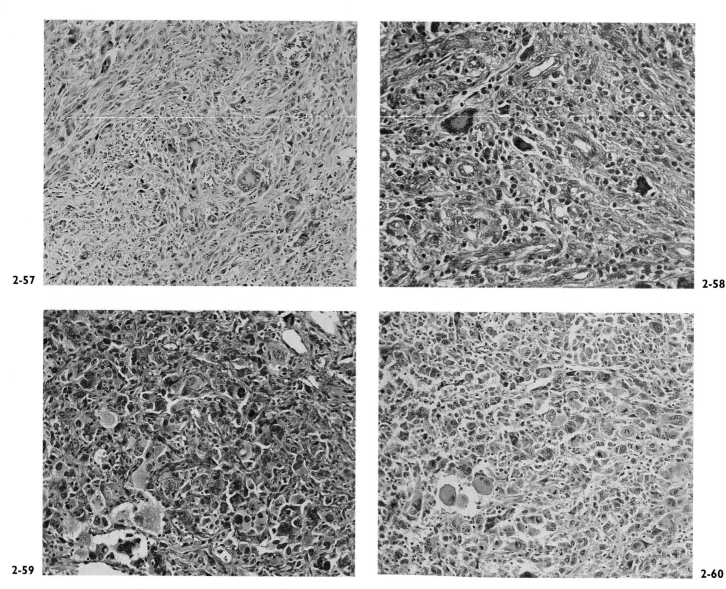

2-57

2-58

2-59

2-60

Figs. 2-57 through 2-66 Various examples of pleomorphic MFH displaying bizarre cells and a less conspicuous storiform pattern. Some of the giant cells are vacuolated due to the presence of lipid. Other cells may be multinucleated, Touton-like, epithelioid with abundant eosinophilic cytoplasm, or spindled. Atypical mitotic figures, scattered inflammatory cells, and a variable amount of collagen may also be present.

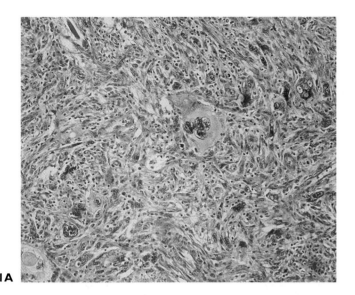

2-61A

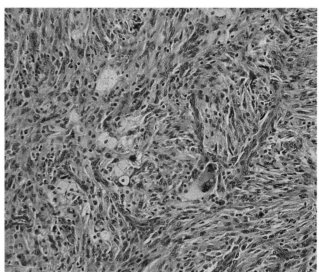

2-61B

Figs. 2-57 through 2-66—cont'd. For legend, see opposite page.

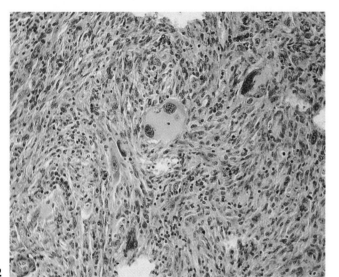

2-62

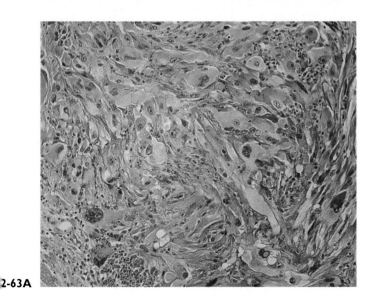

2-63A

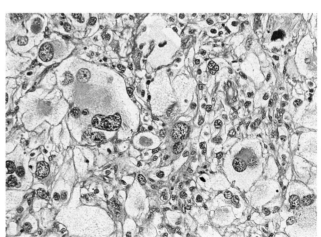

2-63B

(Figs continued on next page.)

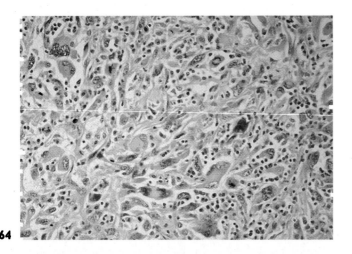

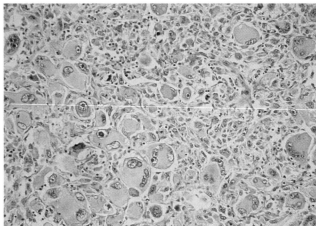

2-64

2-65

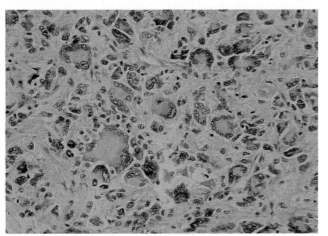

Figs. 2-57 through 2-66—cont'd. For legend, see page 66.

2-66

Myxoid MFH

MICROSCOPIC FEATURES

- >50% myxoid areas
- Conventional MFH areas
- Prominent vasculature
- Perivascular tumor cell growth
- Vacuolated cells (pseudolipoblasts)
- Hyaluronidase sensitive stromal mucin

DIFFERENTIAL DIAGNOSIS

- Nodular fasciitis
- Atypical decubital fibroplasia
- Myxoma
- Myxoid liposarcoma

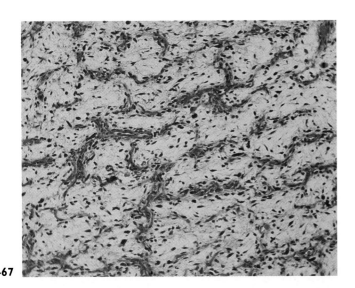

2-67

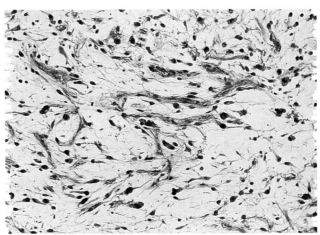

2-68

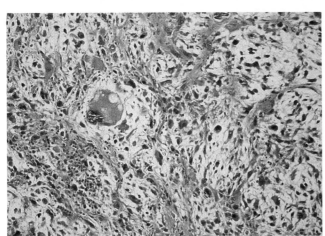

2-69

Figs. 2-67 through 2-69 Typical examples of myxoid MFH of varying grades of malignancy with mild to marked pleomorphism of the spindled cells, an abundant myxoid matrix, and a prominent vascular pattern. Scattered Touton-like or bizarre giant cells, as well as multivacuolated cells containing mucin and simulating lipoblasts, are frequently seen in conjunction with conventional (storiform/pleomorphic) MFH.

Giant Cell MFH

MICROSCOPIC FEATURES

- Multinodular growth pattern
- Conventional MFH areas
- Osteoclast-like giant cells
- Fibroblasts
- Histiocytes
- Focal osteoid (variable)

DIFFERENTIAL DIAGNOSIS

- Fibrous histiocytoma
- Extraskeletal osteosarcoma
- Giant cell tumor of bone with extraosseous extension

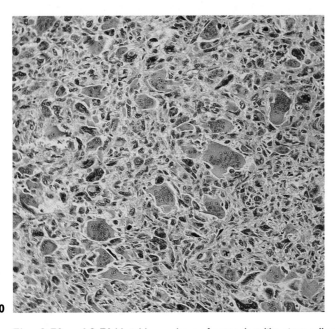

2-70

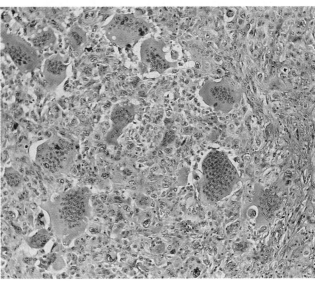

2-71

Figs. 2-70 and 2-71 Variable numbers of osteoclast-like giant cells are seen in the giant cell variant of MFH. Occasionally, asteroid bodies and osteoid may be seen.

Inflammatory MFH

MICROSCOPIC FEATURES

- Xanthoma cells, malignant and benign-appearing
- Secondary inflammation
- Phagocytosis of inflammatory cells
- Conventional MFH areas

DIFFERENTIAL DIAGNOSIS

- Xanthogranulomatous pyelonephritis (extrarenal extension)
- Rosai-Dorfman disease of soft tissue
- Lymphoma (Hodgkin's and non-Hodgkin's)

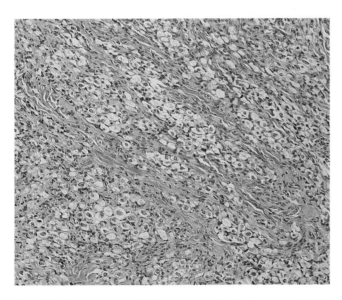

Fig. 2-72 Xanthomatous MFH, a variant of inflammatory MFH, is associated with numerous xanthoma cells with abundant lipid. Rare, bizarre, atypical histiocytoid cells also may be seen.

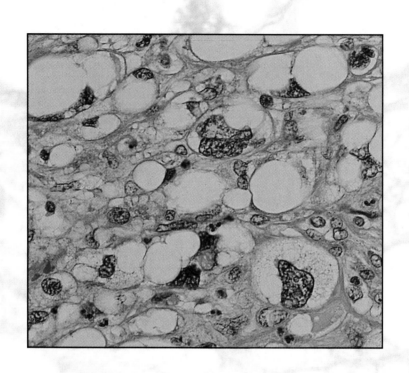

Chapter 3

Lipomatous Tumors

BENIGN

Lipoma

Lipoma is probably the most common mesenchymal neoplasm in humans. It most frequently occurs durring the fifth and sixth decades of life and is more likely to occur in obese individuals. Lipomas are usually divided into cutaneous and deep types. The **cutaneous type** occurs mainly on the back, shoulders, neck, and abdomen and tends to be circumscribed. **Multiple lipomas** account for less than 5% of all lipomas, have a proclivity for the upper trunk, and tend to occur in men in the fifth and sixth decades of life. Familial multiple lipomas and Bannayan-Zonana syndrome (multiple lipomas, macrocephaly, hemangiomas) account for a small proportion of multiple lipomas.

The **deep lipomas** are larger and grossly less well defined than their cutaneous counterparts. Specific types of deep lipoma are distinguished by distinctive clinical and pathologic features and are designated intramuscular, lumbosacral, and perineural lipomas, and lipoma of tendon sheath.

Intramuscular lipomas typically infiltrate the skeletal muscle and fascia of large muscles in the extremities and tend to recur if incompletely excised. **Lipoma of tendon sheath** occurs primarily in young adults in the distal extremities; approximately half are bilateral. In contrast, lipoma arborescens (or hypertrophic synovial villi containing fat) tends to occur in older adults and is associated with chronic arthritis.

Lumbosacral lipoma occurs primarily in children 10 years of age or younger and is associated with spina bifida and not infrequently a lipoma of the spinal cord. Females are affected more than males, and the lesion is associated with progressive myelopathy or radiculopathy in two thirds of cases.

Fibrolipomatous hamartoma of nerve (neural fibrolipoma, perineural lipoma) is a fibrous and fatty growth surrounding and infiltrating large peripheral nerves and their branches, primarily in the distal upper extremities. About one third of cases are associated with macrodactyly and fatty overgrowth. Most patients have had a lesion since birth, and nearly all present before the age of 30 years with symptoms referable to nerve compression.

MICROSCOPIC FEATURES

- Thin capsule (variable)
- Infiltrative growth pattern (intramuscular and lumbosacral lipomas, neural fibrolipoma)
- Mature fat
- Thin fibrous septa
- Atrophy of indigenous tissue (e.g., skeletal muscle, peripheral nerve)
- Myxoid change (variable)
- Chondro-osseous metaplasia (rare)
- Neuroglia, ependymal elements, smooth muscle (lumbosacral lipoma)
- Secondary fat necrosis
- Secondary hemorrhage

DIFFERENTIAL DIAGNOSIS

- Myxoma
- Intramuscular hemangioma with fatty overgrowth
- Atypical lipoma
- Well-differentiated liposarcoma
- Myxoid liposarcoma

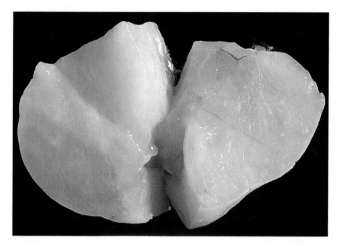

Fig. 3-1 Gross picture of lipoma showing characteristic lobulated pattern.

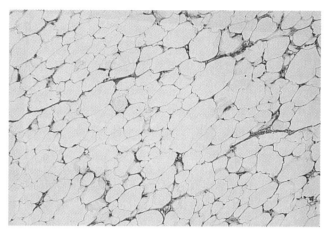

Fig. 3-2 Lipoma composed of lipocytes with peripherally placed, small compressed nuclei.

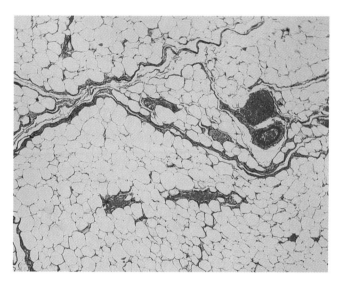

Fig. 3-3 Trichrome stain of lipoma accentuating interlobular fibrous septa and dilated vascular channels.

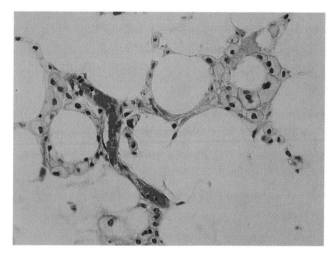

Fig. 3-4 Focal fat necrosis in lipoma with lipophages and scattered chronic inflammatory cells.

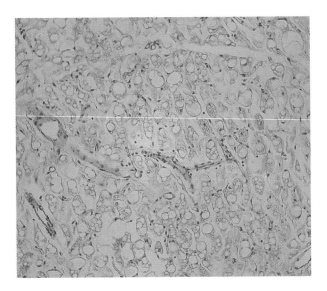

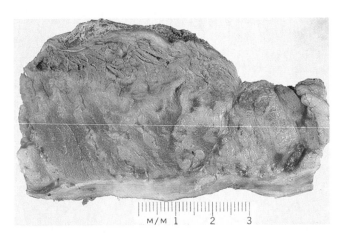

Fig. 3-6 Diffuse infiltration of muscle by mature fat is seen in this gross specimen of an intramuscular lipoma.

Fig. 3-5 Severe fatty atrophy marked by multivacuolated fat cells with small indistinct nuclei, a prominent myxoid matrix, and small vessels.

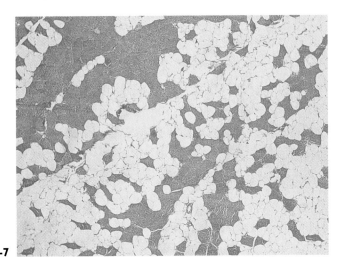

3-7

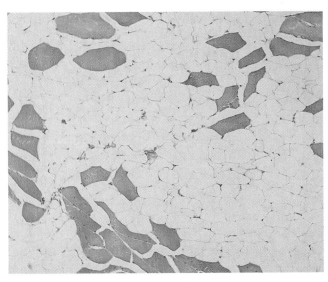

3-8

Figs. 3-7 and 3-8 Characteristic microscopic picture of intramuscular lipoma revealing intimate mixture of proliferating lipocytes and unaltered or slightly atrophic residual striated muscle cells.

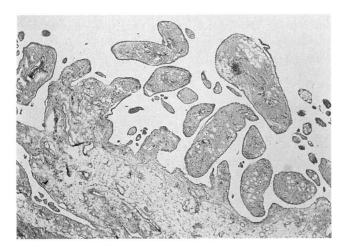

Fig. 3-9 Synovial lipoma ("lipoma arborescens") showing proliferation of fat within synovial villi and subsynovial tissue.

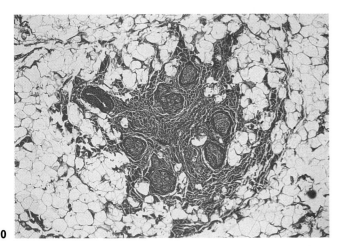

3-10

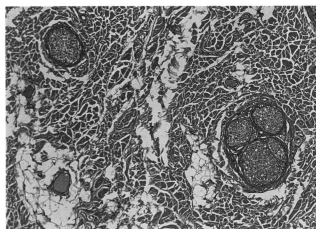

3-11

Figs. 3-10 and 3-11 Neural fibrolipoma (fibrolipomatous hamartoma of nerves); nerve fibers in cross section with perineural fibrofatty growth.

Lipomatosis

Lipomatosis is a localized overgrowth of mature adipose tissue that involves not only the subcutis, but also the underlying musculature, and occasionally, adjacent viscera or organs. The three primary types of lipomatosis are based principally on anatomic location, patient age at presentation, and associated conditions.

Diffuse lipomatosis is extremely rare and consists of a massive overgrowth of mature fat in a large area of the body such as the trunk or an extremity. It usually begins in early childhood and is characterized by rapid growth and multiple recurrences. There may be associated osseous hypertrophy, but

usually no involvement of peripheral nerves. Some cases may be associated with multiple lipomas or angiomas elsewhere in the body.

Cervical symmetric lipomatosis (Madelung's disease) afflicts middle-aged men with a history of ethanol consumption or hepatic disease. Its most outstanding feature is extensive fatty growth about the entire neck, which has been likened to a horse collar. The fatty involvement may extend into the cheeks, breasts, upper arms, axillae, mediastinum, and larynx, potentially causing compression of vital structures. The disease course usually remits with cessation of imbibition and correction of the patient's nutritional status.

Pelvic lipomatosis occurs chiefly in young to middle-aged black men and consists of an overgrowth of mature adipose tissue in the perirectal and perivesical regions that ultimately may cause hydonephrosis with uremia or gastrointestinal tract obstruction if not surgically corrected. There may be an association with multiple lipomas.

MICROSCOPIC FEATURES

- Mature adipose tissue
- Infiltrative growth pattern
- Fibrosis (variable)
- Calcification (rare)

DIFFERENTIAL DIAGNOSIS

- Intramuscular lipoma
- Angiomatosis with fatty overgrowth
- Hemangioma with fatty overgrowth
- Lipoblastomatosis
- Dercum's disease (adiposis dolorosa)
- Well-differentiated liposarcoma

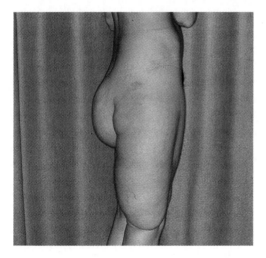

Fig. 3-12 Marked fatty overgrowth in buttock and thigh is seen in this case of diffuse lipomatosis.

Angiolipoma

Angiolipomas are painful subcutaneous lesions that usually occur in young adults, most commonly in the forearm, followed by the trunk and upper arm. Multiple lesions are found in approximately two thirds of cases. No more than 5% of cases are familial.

MICROSCOPIC FEATURES

- Circumscription
- Mature adipose tissue
- Prominent, small, branching vessels
- Fibrin thrombi (diagnostic)
- Perivascular fibrosis (variable)

DIFFERENTIAL DIAGNOSIS

- Lipoma
- Spindle cell lipoma

- Kaposi's sarcoma
- Angiosarcoma

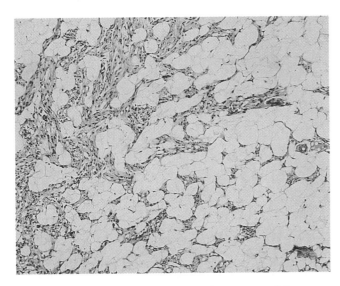

Fig. 3-13 Characteristic angiolipoma with numerous delicate vascular channels associated with spindle cells within mature fat.

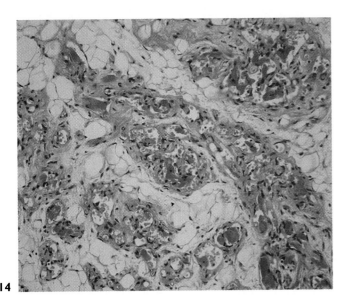

3-14

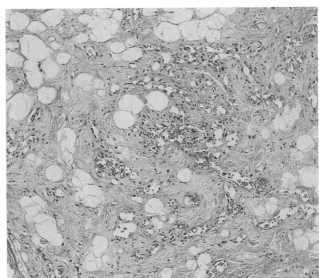

3-15

Figs. 3-14 and 3-15 Angiolipoma with partial replacement of fatty tissue by fibrosis. Occlusion of vascular channels by multiple microthrombi is a characteristic feature of angiolipoma.

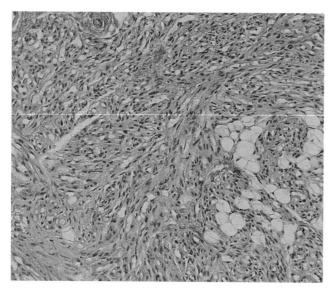

Fig. 3-16 Cellular variant of angiolipoma marked by prominent proliferation of spindle-shaped endothelial cells.

Spindle Cell Lipoma

Spindle cell lipoma is a distinctive, benign fatty tumor that presents as a painless, slow-growing, well-defined, solitary mass most commonly, but not exclusively, occurring in men over 40 years old. The most frequent location is the subcutis of the shoulder and the posterior neck regions, although it also may occur in other locations.

MICROSCOPIC FEATURES

- Circumscribed
- Mature fat
- Uniform, undifferentiated, spindle cells
- Collagen
- Myxoid matrix (variable)
- Mast cells

DIFFERENTIAL DIAGNOSIS

- Myxoma
- Myxolipoma
- Angiolipoma
- Spindle cell liposarcoma
- Myxoid liposarcoma
- Myxoid fibrosarcoma
- Myxoid malignant fibrous histiocytoma

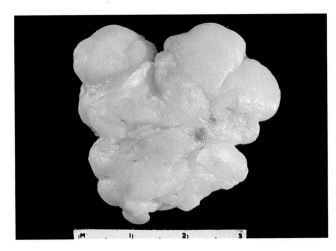

Fig. 3-17 Spindle cell lipoma grossly resembles a lipoma but usually has a more prominent pale staining, glistening cut surface.

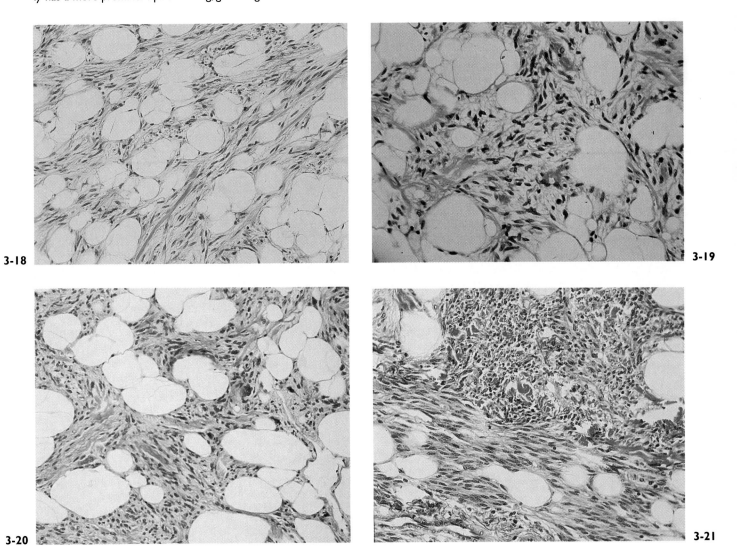

3-18

3-19

3-20

3-21

Figs. 3-18 through 3-22 Typical examples of spindle cell lipoma composed of a variable mixture of mature fat cells and well-oriented, small spindle cells associated with a myxoid matrix and collagen bundles. Mast cells also may be present.

(Figs continued on next page.)

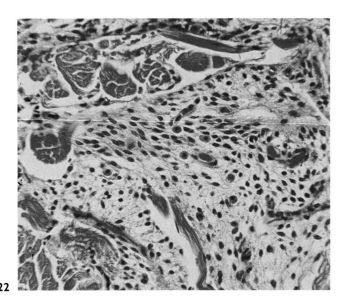

3-22

Figs. 3-18 through 3-22—cont'd. For legend, see page 81.

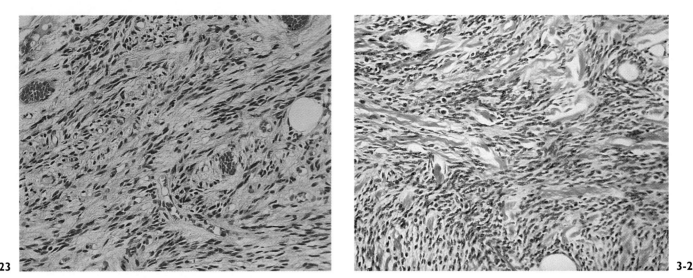

3-23

3-24

Figs. 3-23 and 3-24 Cellular variants of spindle cell lipoma. The subcutaneous location, the circumscription of the lesion, and the lack of cellular pleomorphism help to distinguish it from fibrosarcoma.

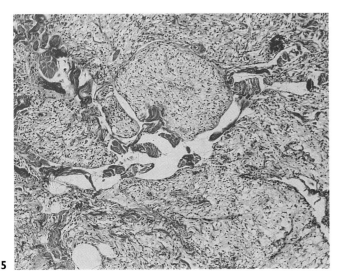

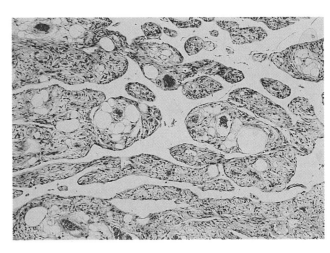

3-25

3-26

Figs. 3-25 and 3-26 Richly vascular pattern in otherwise typical examples of spindle cell lipoma, a feature that may cause confusion with a vascular tumor.

Pleomorphic Lipoma

Pleomorphic lipoma is closely related to, if not, a pleomorphic variant of spindle cell lipoma, as demonstrated by the presence of transitional lesions with features of both classic spindle cell lipoma and pleomorphic lipoma and similar clinical settings. Pleomorphic lipoma is usually well circumscribed and is found primarily in the subcutis of the posterior neck and shoulder region of men 40 years of age or older. Local recurrences are extremely unusual.

MICROSCOPIC FEATURES

- Circumscription
- Multinucleated giant cells (floret cells)
- Collagen and sclerosis
- Lipoblasts (rare)
- Atypical mitoses (rare)
- Myxoid change (variable)
- Chronic inflammation

DIFFERENTIAL DIAGNOSIS

- Atypical lipoma
- Sclerosing well-differentiated liposarcoma
- Pleomorphic liposarcoma
- Malignant fibrous histiocytoma

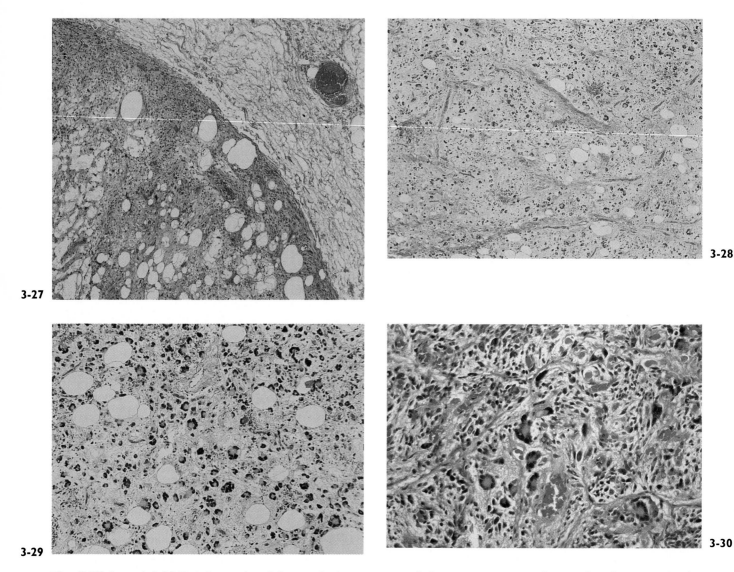

3-27

3-28

3-29

3-30

Figs. 3-27 through 3-30 Typical examples of pleomorphic lipoma composed of an intimate mixture of mature fat cells, scattered multi-nucleated giant cells with eosinophilic cytoplasm and peripherally placed wreathlike nuclei (floret cells), a myxoid matrix, and broad bundles of collagen. Fig. 3-27 shows sharp circumscription of lesion.

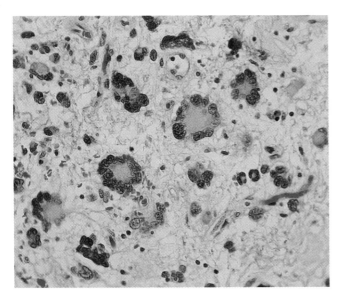

Fig. 3-31 Characteristic floret-type giant cells of pleomorphic lipoma displaying a deeply eosinophilic cytoplasm and multiple, peripherally placed rounded nuclei.

Myolipoma

This benign neoplasm is composed of well-differentiated, benign adipose tissue and smooth muscle. The most common location described thus far is the trunk, including the retroperitoneum, abdominal cavity and abdominal wall, and inguinal region; lesions on the back and leg also have been noted. A relationship to angiomyolipoma or tuberous sclerosis has not been identified.

MICROSCOPIC FEATURES

- Partial encapsulation
- Mature adipose tissue
- Benign smooth muscle fascicles
- Sclerosis (variable)

DIFFERENTIAL DIAGNOSIS

- Leiomyoma
- Leiomyosarcoma
- Liposarcoma with smooth muscle differentiation

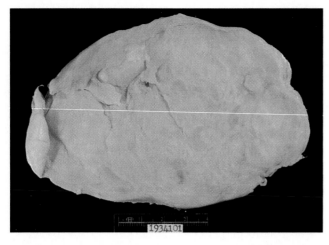

Fig. 3-32 Gross picture of myolipoma showing mixture of fat and gray-white (smooth muscle) tissue.

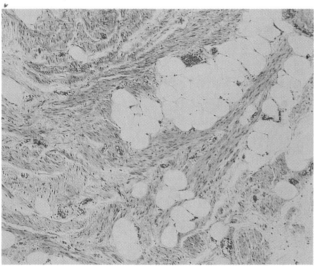

3-33

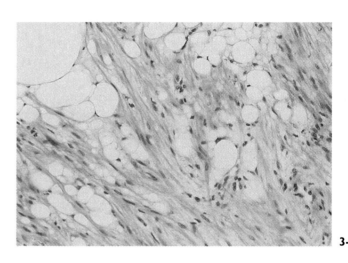

3-34

Figs. 3-33 and 3-34 Typical myolipoma composed of mature fat cells separated by bundles of well-differentiated smooth muscle.

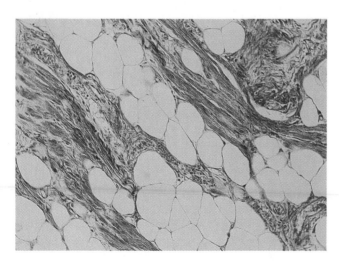

Fig. 3-35 Trichrome stain of myolipomas revealing combination of fuchsinophilic smooth muscle fibers, lipocytes, and fibrous tissue.

Angiomyolipoma

Angiomyolipoma is a hamartomatous lesion, usually occurring either within or intimately associated with the kidney; pedunculated or satellite nodules may be found in the adjacent soft tissue and, less commonly, in regional lymph nodes. Similar lesions have also been found in the liver and mediastinum. Approximately one third to one half of cases are associated with tuberous sclerosis; less rarely they are associated with lymphangiomyoma and lymphangiomyomatosis. Solitary forms are more common than bilateral lesions; the latter are more often associated with tuberous sclerosis. They occur more frequently in women than men. They may be asymptomatic or cause abdominal pain, fever and chills, hematuria, or massive hemorrhage secondary to rupture.

MICROSCOPIC FEATURES

- Variable proportions of
  1. Mature adipose tissue (may be mildly pleomorphic)
  2. Medium-sized vessels with thick walls and no elastic lamina
  3. Irregular bundles of smooth muscle (may be pleomorphic)
- Extramedullary hematopoiesis (rare)
- Intravascular growth (rare)

DIFFERENTIAL DIAGNOSIS

- Leiomyoma
- Leiomyosarcoma
- Liposarcoma

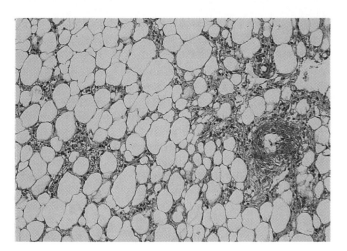

Fig. 3-36 Typical microscopic picture of angiomyolipoma consisting of lipocytes and medium-sized, thick-walled vessels. Smooth muscle is present elsewhere in the lesion.

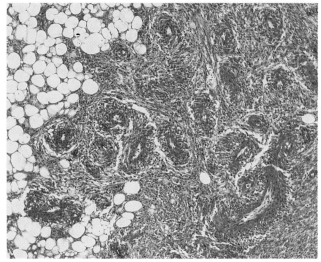

Fig. 3-37 Cellular variant of angiomyolipoma marked by the presence of rounded, eosinophilic cells with plump nuclei (modified smooth muscle elements) and mature fat cells.

Myelolipoma

This hamartomatous lesion usually occurs in the adrenal gland, but may also occur in the retroperitoneal and pelvic soft tissues. Patients are usually 40 years of age or older at presentation; large tumors may be symptomatic, but several are incidental findings at surgery or autopsy. In general these are solitary masses. On rare occasions, multicentric lesions may also be seen. These may be associated with disturbances of adrenocortical metabolism and are not typically associated with myelophthisic processes or malignant hematopoietic proliferations.

MICROSCOPIC FEATURES

- Bone marrow elements
- Mature fat

DIFFERENTIAL DIAGNOSIS

- Extramedullary hematopoiesis
- Lipoma

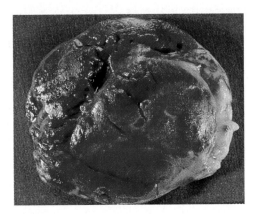

Fig. 3-38 Gross picture of myelolipoma.

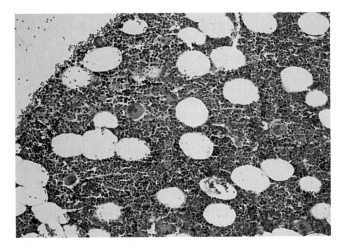

Fig. 3-39 Myelolipoma showing typical mixture of bone marrow elements and fat cells.

Hibernoma

Hibernomas tend to occur in young adults, primarily in the scapular region, although the chest wall, back, thigh, and inguinal and axillary regions may also be affected. Typically, this slow-growing, painless mass is cured by complete excision. Intermediate forms between lipoma and hibernoma, with a prominent component of mature adult adipose tissue, are probably more common than pure hibernomas.

MICROSCOPIC FEATURES

- Lobular pattern
- Granular to multivacuolated eosinophilic cytoplasm
- Round to oval cells
- Centrally located nuclei
- Golden-brown cytoplasmic pigment (liposfuscin)
- Mature fat

DIFFERENTIAL DIAGNOSIS

- Adult rhabdomyoma
- Granular cell tumor
- Round cell liposarcoma

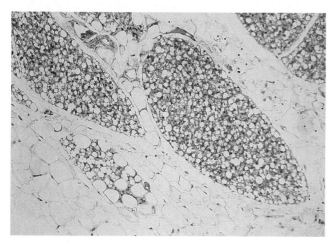

Fig. 3-40 Remnants of well-circumscribed lobules of brown fat within periadrenal fat.

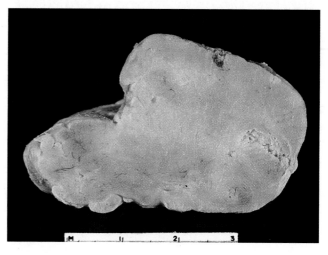

Fig. 3-41 Gross picture of hibernoma showing typical yellow to orange color of the lesion.

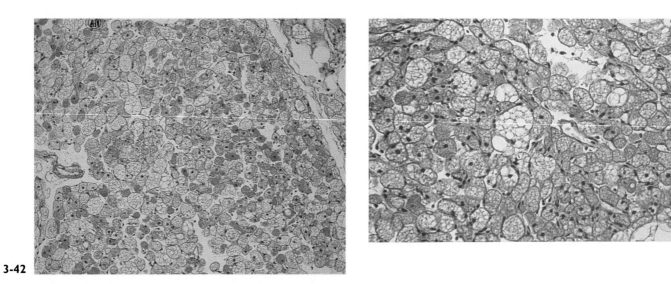

3-42

3-43

Figs. 3-42 and 3-43 Typical examples of hibernoma consisting of multivacuolated brown fat cells having small, rounded nuclei.

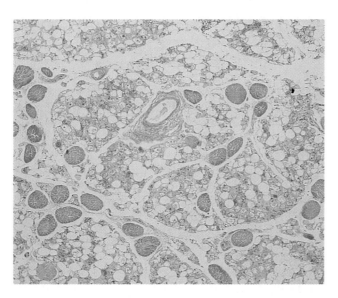

Fig. 3-44 Typical hibernoma growing within striated muscle.

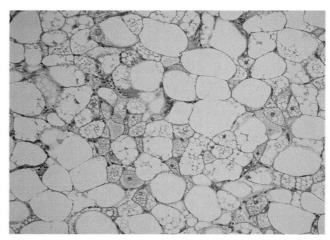

Fig. 3-45 Hibernoma: higher magnification demonstrating brown fat cells in varying stages of differentiation ranging from eosinophilic cells and multivacuolated cells to mature fat cells.

Lipoblastoma

This variant of lipoma occurs in children, primarily those 3 years of age or younger. Both localized and diffuse forms exist and are referred to as lipoblastoma and lipoblastomatosis, respectively. Whereas lipoblastoma usually is confined to the subcutis, lipoblastomatosis diffusely infiltrates groups of skeletal muscles, as well as the subcutis. Males are affected twice as commonly as females. Lipoblastoma typically involves the upper or lower limbs. Recurrences are seen primarily with the diffuse form of disease. Sequential biopsies of lipoblastoma show eventual maturation to adult-type fat.

MICROSCOPIC FEATURES

- Distinct lobular architecture
- Fibrous septa
- Myxoid matrix (variable)
- Mast cells (variable)

- Immature fat composed of the following:
  1. Stellate or primitive spindled cells
  2. Univacuolated and multivacuolated lipoblasts
  3. Hibernoma-like areas (variable)

DIFFERENTIAL DIAGNOSIS

- Lipoma
- Lipomatosis

- Spindle cell lipoma
- Myxoid liposarcoma

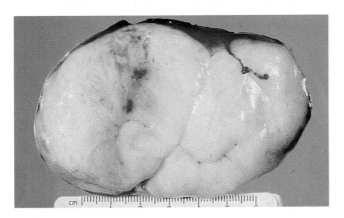

Fig. 3-46 Typical gross picture of a lipoblastoma involving the right lower leg of a 2-year-old infant. The lesion is well circumscribed, lobulated, and has a glistening cut surface.

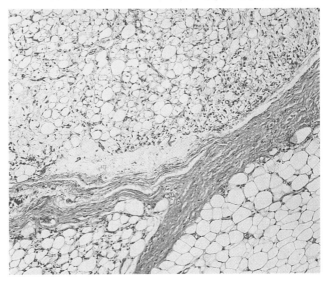

Fig. 3-47 Low-magnification picture of lipoblastoma exhibiting characteristic multilobular pattern.

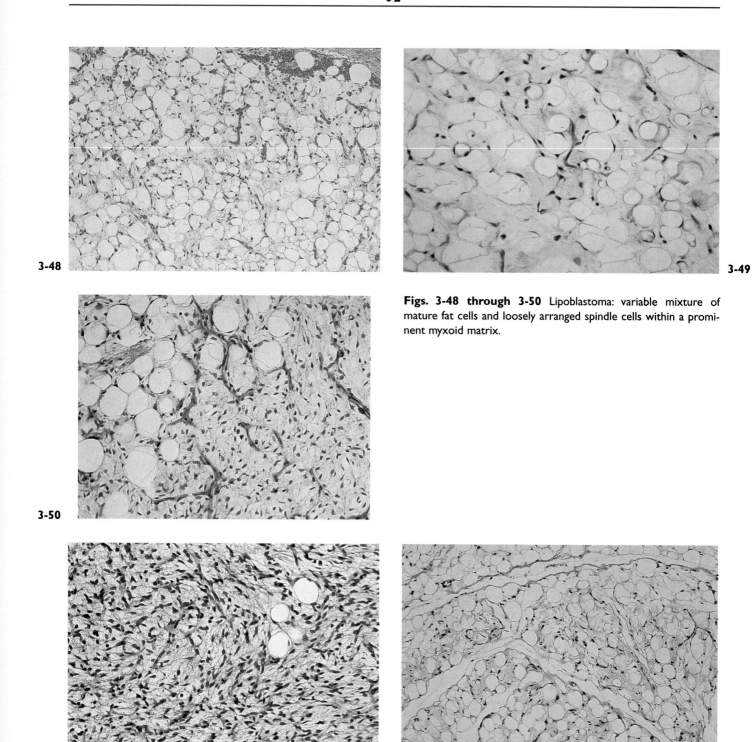

3-48

3-49

Figs. 3-48 through 3-50 Lipoblastoma: variable mixture of mature fat cells and loosely arranged spindle cells within a prominent myxoid matrix.

3-50

3-51A

3-51B

Fig. 3-51 A, B Lipoblastoma: progressive maturation of tumor in two consecutive biopsies 1 year apart.

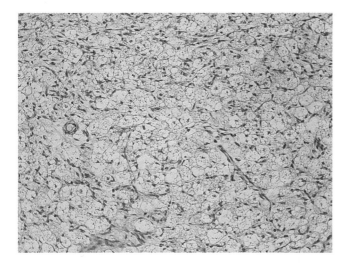

Fig. 3-52 Hibernoma-like lipoblastoma composed of numerous multivacuolated fat cells of uniform appearance.

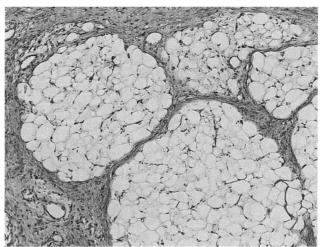

Fig. 3-53 Lipoblastomatosis: lobular pattern and separation of individual lobules by fibrous trabeculae.

BORDERLINE

Atypical Lipoma

Atypical lipoma is a term that has been used in place of well-differentiated liposarcoma (both the sclerosing and lipoma-like variants) when it occurs in the subcutis and muscle of the extremities or superficial tissues of the trunk. The intent of using this term is to prevent unnecessarily radical surgery for an intrinsically low-grade neoplasm. Morphologically, it is indistinguishable from some well-differentiated liposarcomas at other sites.

MICROSCOPIC FEATURES

■ See Well-Differentiated Liposarcoma.

DIFFERENTIAL DIAGNOSIS

■ See Well-Differentiated Liposarcoma.

MALIGNANT

Liposarcoma

Liposarcoma is one of the most common sarcomas of adults and occurs primarily in the fifth through seventh decades of life. Occurrence in children is rare. Sites commonly involved include the thigh, retroperitoneum, inguinal region, and spermatic cord. The four major histologic types of liposarcoma are well differentiated, myxoid and round cell, pleomorphic, and dedifferentiated. Spindle cell variants of liposarcoma are also recognized. Histologic subclassification is prognostically significant. Well-differentiated and myxoid liposarcomas behave in a low-grade fashion and are characterized by multiple local recurrences, a lower metastatic rate, and a more protracted clinical course than the high-grade liposarcomas, which include dedifferentiated, pleomorphic, and round cell types. The latter three liposarcomas behave more aggressively and are associated with a shorter survival and pulmonary and visceral metastases. Occasional mixed types of liposarcoma are not easily classified. Tumor location is also important in prognosis, and some types of liposarcoma have a propensity for certain locations. Superficial and intramuscular lesions are more amenable to complete excision than deep-seated lesions of the retroperitoneum, mediastinum, or inguinal/paratesticular region.

Well-Differentiated Liposarcoma

This type of liposarcoma includes the **lipoma-like** and **sclerosing** subtypes of **liposarcoma**. They are found most commonly in the thigh, retroperitoneum, and paratesticular/inguinal region.

MICROSCOPIC FEATURES

- Mature fat
- Enlarged, hyperchromatic, peripheral nuclei
- Lipoblasts
- Giant cells with peripherally oriented nuclei and abundant, eosinophilic cytoplasm (floret cells)
- Fibrous septa
- Chronic inflammatory cells
- Myxoid stroma (variable)
- Smooth muscle differentiation (rare)

DIFFERENTIAL DIAGNOSIS

- Fat necrosis
- Myxoid change in benign fat (myxolipoma)
- Lipogranuloma
- Panniculitis
- Hibernoma
- Lipomatosis
- Pleomorphic lipoma
- Myxoid liposarcoma
- Dedifferentiated liposarcoma
- Pleomorphic liposarcoma

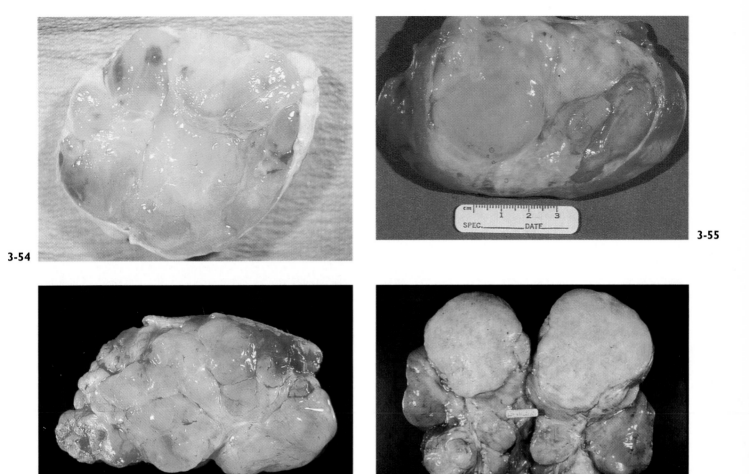

3-54

3-55

3-56

3-57

Figs. 3-54 through 3-57 Various gross pictures of liposarcoma.

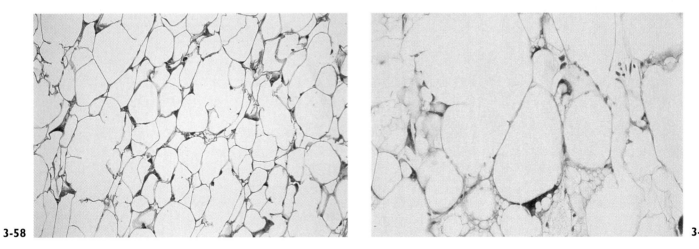

3-58

3-59

Figs. 3-58 through 3-60 Microscopic pictures of well-differentiated liposarcomas displaying a mixture of mature fat cells and lipoblasts with hyperchromatic, atypical nuclei.

(Figs continued on next page.)

Lipomatous Tumors

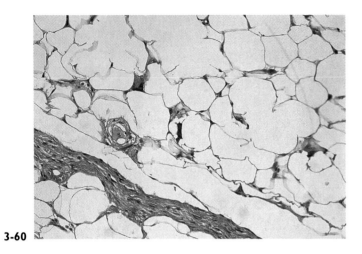

Figs. 3-58 through 3-60—cont'd. For legend, see page 95.

3-60

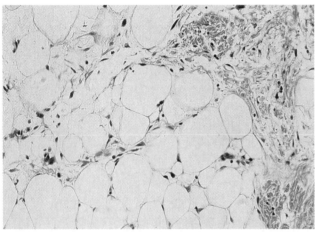

3-61

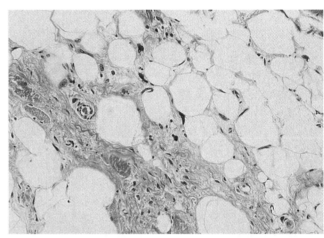

3-62

Figs. 3-61 through 3-63 Well-differentiated liposarcoma with scattered atypical spindle cells; some are located within fibrous trabecula.

3-63

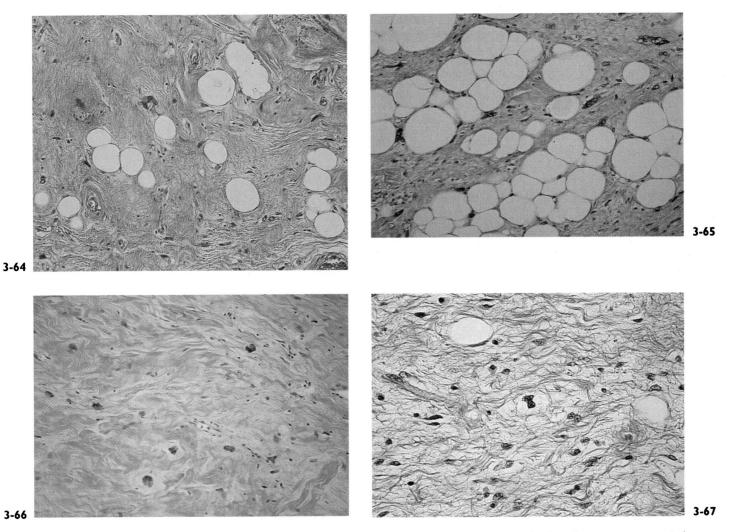

Figs. 3-64 through 3-67 Typical examples of slerosing (fibrosing) liposarcoma demonstrating scattered cells with one or more atypical nuclei within a predominantly fibrous stroma.

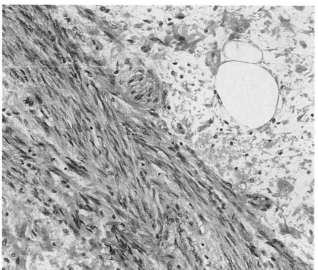

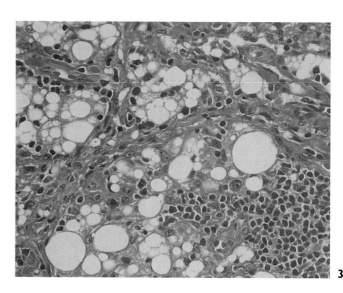

3-68A   3-68B

Fig. 3-68 A, Well-differentiated liposarcoma with smooth muscle differentiation. **B,** Sclerosing lipogranuloma simulating liposarcoma. Lipophages often closely resemble lipoblasts, but in general show little or no nuclear atypism and usually are associated with inflammatory elements, including plasma cells.

Myxoid and Round Cell Liposarcoma

Myxoid and round cell liposarcoma tend to occur in the limbs and limb girdles and are capable of multiple local recurrences and metastases.

Round cell liposarcoma (cellular myxoid liposarcoma) is considered to be a poorly differentiated myxoid liposarcoma, which behaves as a high-grade liposarcoma.

MICROSCOPIC FEATURES

- Multilobular architecture
- Univacuolated and multivacuolated lipoblasts
- Hibernoma-like lipoblasts
- Primitive round to angulated cells
- Spindled cells (rare)
- Myxoid matrix (hyaluronidase sensitive)

- Adult fat (variable)
- Giant cells (rare)
- Adenoid or cording pattern (rare)
- Cystic spaces
- Hemorrhage
- Chondro-osseous differentiation (rare)

DIFFERENTIAL DIAGNOSIS

- Spindle cell lipoma with myxoid change
- Hibernoma
- Angiolipoma
- Lipoblastoma
- Myxoma

- Angiomyxoma
- Myxoid dermatofibrosarcoma protuberans
- Myxoid malignant fibrous histiocytoma
- Signet ring lymphoma
- Ewing's sarcoma

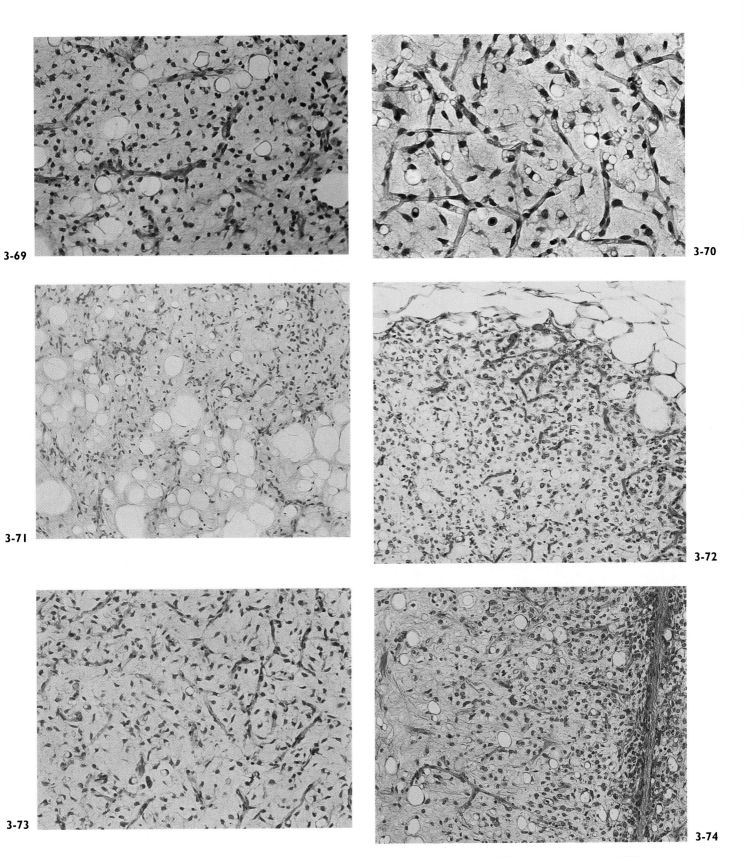

3-69

3-70

3-71

3-72

3-73

3-74

Figs. 3-69 through 3-74 Typical examples of myxoid liposarcoma. The tumor is composed of lipoblasts in various stages of differentiation, ranging from primitive mesenchymal cells to well-differentiated lipoblasts, a delicate plexiform capillary pattern, and abundant myxoid stroma.

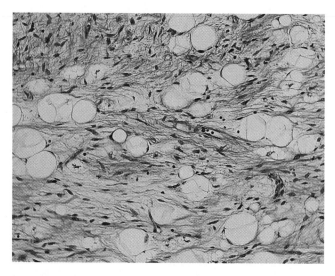

Fig. 3-75 Variant of myxoid liposarcoma showing a prominent spindle cell pattern and interspersed lipoblasts: spindle cell liposarcoma.

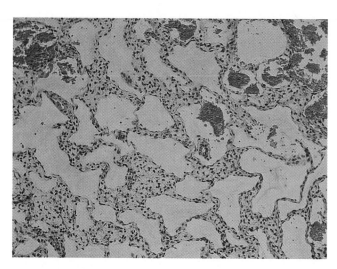

Fig. 3-76 Myxoid liposarcoma with prominent vascular pattern simulating a vascular tumor.

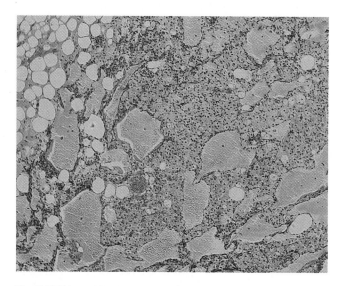

Fig. 3-77 Myxoid liposarcoma marked by pools of myxoid material.

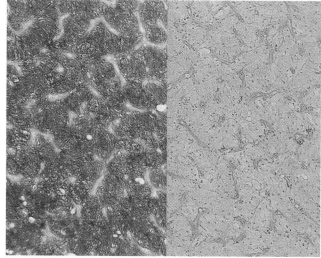

Fig. 3-78 Colloidal iron stain with and without hyaluronidase revealing abundant hyaluronidase-sensitive mucoid material, lipid-containing lipoblasts, and a distinct capillary pattern.

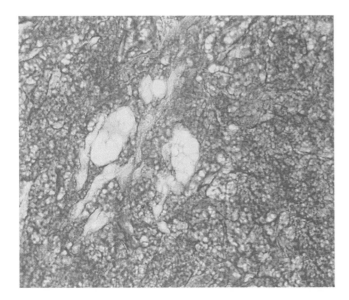

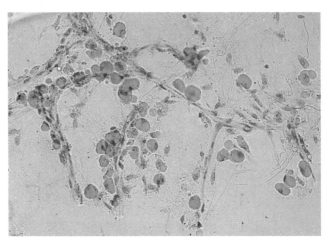

Fig. 3-80 Oil-red-O (ORO) fat stain of myxoid liposarcoma showing scattered ORO-positive lipoblasts.

Fig. 3-79 Colloidal iron stain of myxoid liposarcoma staining the mucoid matrix between the lipoblasts and vessels a deep blue color.

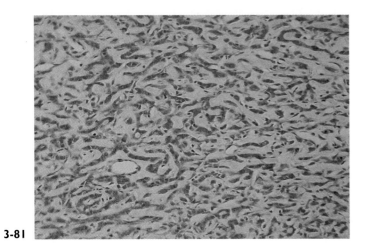

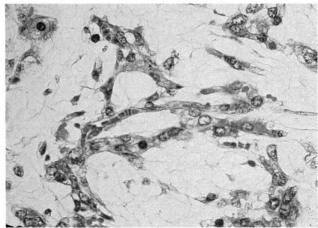

3-81

3-82

Figs. 3-81 and 3-82 Myxoid liposarcoma with focal cording of tumor cells.

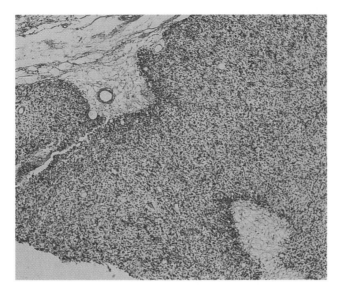

Fig. 3-83 Round cell liposarcoma (poorly differentiated myxoid liposarcoma) consisting of sheets of small, rounded tumor cells.

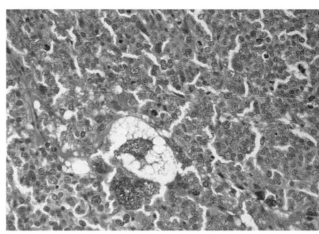

Fig. 3-84 Round cell liposarcoma showing single, large multivacuolated lipoblast. Note characteristic scalloped nucleus.

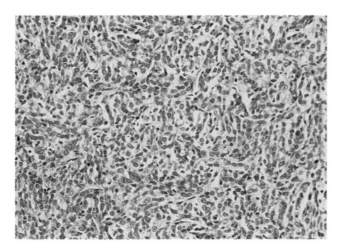

Fig. 3-85 Round cell liposarcoma demonstrating distinct cording of tumor cells.

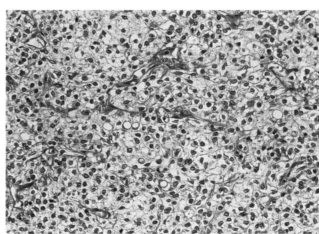

Fig. 3-86 Round cell liposarcoma with scattered signet-ring-shaped lipoblasts.

Pleomorphic Liposarcoma

This high-grade liposarcoma with metastatic potential occurs chiefly in the limbs and limb girdles. It is usually deep-seated but may be superficial.

MICROSCOPIC FEATURES

- Bizarre, giant lipoblasts
- Xanthoma-like lipoblasts, sometimes numerous
- Malignant fibrous histiocytoma–like foci
- Fibrosis
- Hemorrhage
- Necrosis

DIFFERENTIAL DIAGNOSIS

- Sclerotic pleomorphic lipoma
- Well-differentiated sclerosing liposarcoma
- Myxoid malignant fibrous histiocytoma
- Malignant fibrous histiocytoma

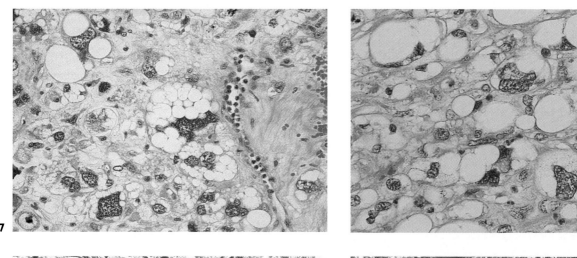

3-87

3-88

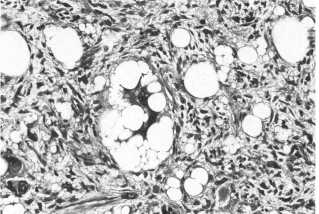

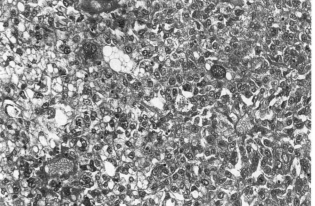

3-89

3-90

Figs. 3-87 through 3-90 Pleomorphic liposarcoma: the lesion is composed of multiple lipoblasts in varying shapes and sizes and poorly differentiated tumor cells without evidence of lipoblastic differentiation.

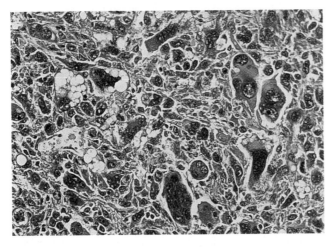

Fig. 3-91 Liposarcoma with pleomorphic lipoblasts and pleomorphic spindle cells.

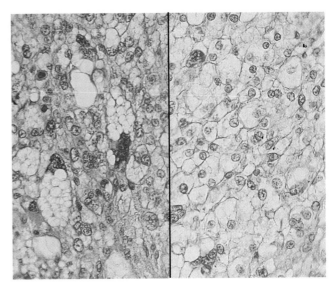

Fig. 3-92 Variant of pleomorphic liposarcoma with lipoblastic and clear cell features.

Dedifferentiated Liposarcoma

These liposarcomas are bimorphic with well-differentiated liposarcoma juxtaposed to a high-grade sarcomatous element such as malignant fibrous histiocytoma or fibrosarcoma. They typically occur in the retroperitoneum, paratesticular region, and to a much lesser extent, in the extremities.

MICROSCOPIC FEATURES

- Malignant fibrous histiocytoma or fibrosarcomatous areas (confluent foci)
- Well-differentiated liposarcoma

DIFFERENTIAL DIAGNOSIS

- Malignant fibrous histiocytoma
- Fibrosarcoma
- Pleomorphic liposarcoma

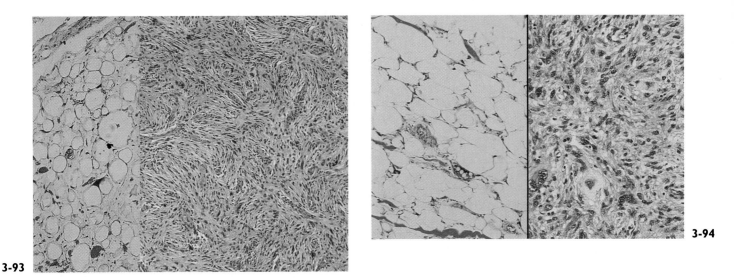

Figs. 3-93 and 3-94 Dedifferentiated liposarcoma with both well-differentiated and poorly differentiated components in different portions of the tumor.

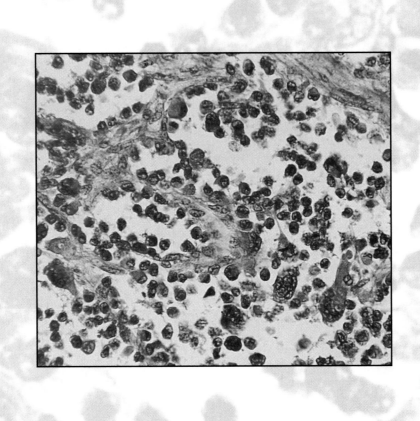

Chapter 4

Myogenic Tumors

SMOOTH MUSCLE: BENIGN

Leiomyoma

Leiomyomas of soft tissue can be divided into cutaneous or superficial leiomyoma, angiomyoma (vascular leiomyoma), and deep leiomyoma. Although smooth muscle proliferations arising along the peritoneal surface (leiomyomatosis peritonealis disseminata) and the pelvic or uterine vasculature (intravenous leiomyomatosis) are not soft tissue tumors per se, they are included because they could be confused with leiomyosarcoma.

muscles and those arising in the genital region. The former compose approximately 75% of all cutaneous leiomyomas, occur primarily along the extensor surfaces of the extremities in young adults, and are usually multiple, slow-growing, and painful. Their multiplicity may make complete excision difficult and probably accounts for a local recurrence rate approaching 50%. Genital leiomyomas, in contrast, are uncommon, solitary masses that average about 2 cm and occur in the nipple, scrotum, labia, and penis.

Cutaneous Leiomyoma

There are essentially two types of cutaneous leiomyoma: those arising from the pilar arrector

MICROSCOPIC FEATURES

- Irregular, ill-defined margins (pilar type)
- Association with hair follicle (pilar type)
- Circumscribed (genital type)
- Mitoses absent
- Atrophic epidermis
- Grenz zone

- Well-differentiated smooth muscle displaying:
  1. Spindled cells with eosinophilic and fuchsinophilic, longitudinal myofibrils
  2. Symmetrical, oval, blunt–ended nuclei
  3. Interlacing bundles and fascicles

DIFFERENTIAL DIAGNOSIS

- Fibrous histiocytoma
- Accessory nipple

- Other hamartomas or choristomas
- Leiomyosarcoma

Deep Leiomyoma

This extremely rare lesion occurs almost exclusively in adults. It involves primarily the deep

muscle of the extremities, abdominal cavity, and retroperitoneum.

MICROSCOPIC FEATURES

- Circumscription
- Interlacing fascicles
- Well-differentiated smooth muscle
- Degenerative pleomorphism (pleomorphic leiomyoma)
- Mitoses absent
- Nuclear palisading (rare)

- Paranuclear glycogen vacuoles (variable)
- Clear cell change (rare)
- Fibrosis (variable)
- Calcification (variable)
- Ossification (rare)

DIFFERENTIAL DIAGNOSIS

- Round ligament
- Fibrous histiocytoma
- Leiomyosarcoma

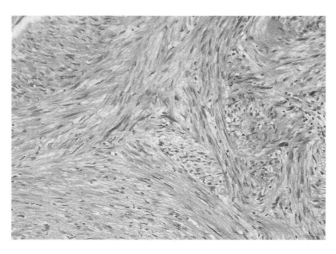

Fig. 4-1 Deep leiomyoma of the popliteal fossa composed of uniform, elongated smooth muscle cells with slight cellular pleomorphism but no mitotic activity.

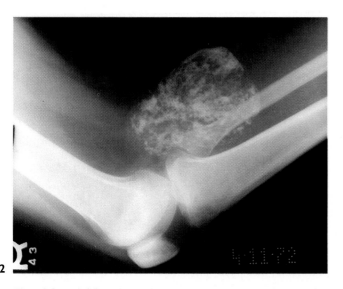

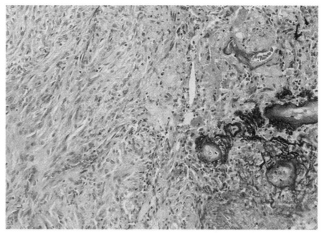

4-2

4-3

Figs. 4-2 and 4-3 Radiographic and microscopic appearance of a deep leiomyoma revealing calcification—a frequent occurrence in long-standing leiomyomas.

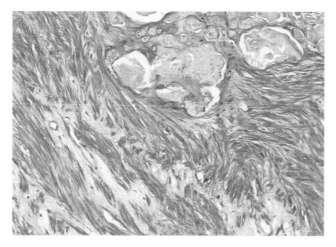

Fig. 4-4 Trichrome stain of deep leiomyoma demonstrating deeply fuchsinophilic spindle cells and focal calcification.

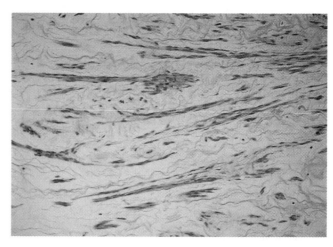

Fig. 4-5 Deep leiomyoma markedly distorted by extensive myxoid change (myxoid leiomyoma).

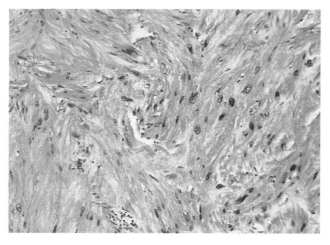

Fig. 4-6 Pleomorphic leiomyoma marked by considerable cellular pleomorphism, but lacking increased mitotic activity or focal necrosis.

Angiomyoma

This unique type of superficial leiomyoma characteristically occurs in the deep dermis or subcutis of women during the fourth through sixth decades of life; it accounts for approximately 25% of super-ficial leiomyomas. Most lesions are less than 2 cm, solitary, and well demarcated and present as a painful mass on the extremities, particularly the lower leg.

MICROSCOPIC FEATURES

- Circumscribed
- Thick-walled, coalescing blood vessels devoid of an internal and external elastic lamina and with partially patent lumina
- Disorganized smooth muscle in the outer vessel wall

- No mitoses
- Hyalinized (variable)
- Calcified (variable)
- Myxoid change (rare)
- Fat between vessels (rare)

DIFFERENTIAL DIAGNOSIS

- Fibroma
- Fibrous histiocytoma
- Leiomyosarcoma

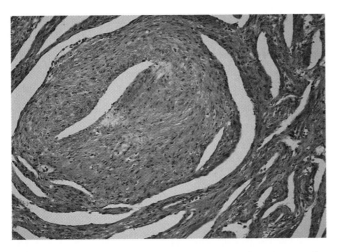

Fig. 4-7 Low magnification of an angiomyoma showing irregular vascular spaces surrounded by deeply eosinophilic, well-differentiated smooth muscle. Note vascular dilation in the capsular region.

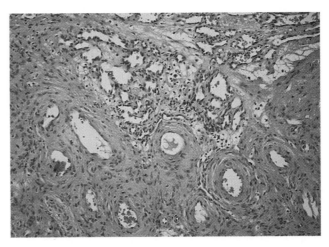

Fig. 4-8 Angiomyoma composed of smooth muscle surrounding vascular channels and cavernous hemangioma–like features at the periphery.

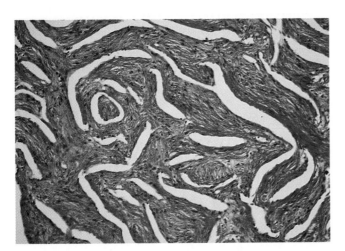

Fig. 4-9 Angiomyoma composed of congeries of small-to-medium-sized, thick-walled vessels surrounded by well-differentiated smooth muscle (trichrome stain).

Intravenous Leiomyomatosis

A rare condition, intravenous leiomyomatosis is characterized by an intravascular growth of benign smooth muscle within the uterine or pelvic veins, either as an extension from a uterine leiomyoma or exclusively within the vessels. It occurs primarily in premenopausal women (over half of whom have had a prior pregnancy) and is frequently associated with uterine leiomyomas. Rare extension into the inferior vena cava, right atrium, and lungs has been documented.

MICROSCOPIC FEATURES

- Intravascular growth
- Variable cellularity
- Round to oval nuclei
- Clear cytoplasm (variable)
- Fibrosis (variable)
- Mitoses (rare)

DIFFERENTIAL DIAGNOSIS

- Benign metastasizing leiomyoma
- Leiomyosarcoma

Leiomyomatosis Peritonealis Disseminata

In this rare subserosal proliferation, multiple smooth muscle nodules have disseminated throughout the peritoneal cavity. It is frequently an incidental finding and has a predilection for pregnant and black women. It is believed to arise from pluripotential cells of the peritoneum, possibly fibroblasts and myofibroblasts, that are hormonally induced to differentiate into smooth muscle and decidualized cells. The lesions regress with removal of estrogen and progesterone and recrudesce with subsequent pregnancy.

MICROSCOPIC FEATURES

- Nodular or permeative subserosal growth pattern
- Fascicles of smooth muscle
- Myofibroblasts
- Decidualized cells (variable)
- Mild nuclear pleomorphism
- Hyalinization (variable)
- Associated endometriosis (rare)
- No hemorrhage or necrosis
- Mitoses (rare)

DIFFERENTIAL DIAGNOSIS

- Decidual reaction
- Leiomyosarcoma
- Mesothelioma

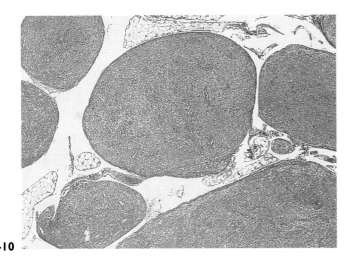

4-10

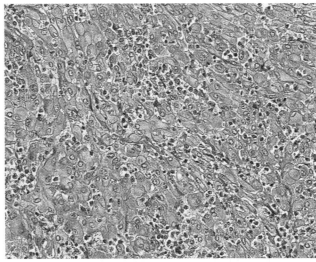

4-11

4-12

Figs. 4-10 through 4-12 Various examples of leiomyomatosis peritonealis disseminata. Decidual change may be seen (Fig. 4-11, from a woman who was 12 weeks pregnant.) Endometriosis may also be associated with leiomyomatosis peritonealis disseminata.

SMOOTH MUSCLE: MALIGNANT

Leiomyosarcoma

The three major categories of leiomyosarcoma in soft tissue, in decreasing frequency, are retroperitoneal and intra-abdominal leiomyosarcoma, cutaneous and subcutantous leiomyosarcoma, and vascular leiomyosarcoma. With the exception of degenerative features that tend to occur in the large retroperitoneal tumors, they have similar histologic features. Anatomic location, which is closely interrelated to tumor depth and size, is by far more important prognostically than histologic features.

Cutaneous and Subcutaneous Leiomyosarcoma

Men are affected two to three times more often than women, usually between the fifth and seventh decades of life. Like cutaneous leiomyoma, cutaneous leiomyosarcoma tends to involve the extensor surfaces of the extremities. Cutaneous lesions are usually ill defined because they merge with the adjacent dermal collagen and pilar arrector muscle, whereas the subcutaneous lesions are well demarcated and larger. Recurrence rates and metastases are related to tumor depth and size. Cutaneous lesions metastasize in 10% of cases or less; in contrast, subcutaneous lesions metastasize in 30% to 40% of cases. Metastases are usually to the lungs and regional lymph nodes.

Retroperitoneal and Intraabdominal Leiomyosarcoma

Approximately two thirds of these lesions occur in women later in life, with the retroperitoneum being the most common site of soft tissue leiomyosarcoma. Symptoms are largely referable to a mass. The most common metastatic sites are the liver and lungs.

Leiomyosarcoma of Vascular Origin

Leiomyosarcoma arising within blood vessels occurs in large veins far more frequently than arteries. The three main vascular sites involved (other than those that arise in the deep veins of the distal extremities) are the inferior vena cava; other veins such as the saphenous, iliac, and femoral veins; and the pulmonary artery. The overwhelming majority of those in the inferior vena cava occur in women, and the prognosis is largely a function of location and surgical accessibility. Leiomyosarcomas occurring in other veins and arteries tend to affect both sexes equally. Those in the extremities may present with edema or evidence of venous occlusion, whereas those in the pulmonary artery are associated with symptoms of pulmonary outflow tract obstruction and right heart failure. Metastases of leiomyosarcomas of vascular origin are frequent and usually to the liver, lymph nodes, lungs, and abdominal organs. In general vascular leiomyosarcomas have an abysmal prognosis.

MICROSCOPIC FEATURES

- Circumscription (deep soft tissue lesions)
- Fascicles that are interlacing or oriented at right angles
- Spindled cells with abundant, fibrillary, eosinophilic cytoplasm
- Symmetric, "cigar"-shaped nuclei
- Atypical nuclear features
- Mitoses (any mitotic activity is suspect for malignancy)
- Paranuclear glycogen vacuoles
- Epithelioid or round cells with clear to vacuolated cytoplasm (rare)
- Hyalinization (variable)
- Necrosis (variable)
- Myxoid change (rare)
- Palisading (rare)
- Multinucleated or osteoclast-like giant cells (rare)
- Malignant fibrous histiocytoma-like foci (variable)

DIFFERENTIAL DIAGNOSIS

- Leiomyoma
- Postoperative (reactive) myofibroblastic nodules
- Malignant peripheral nerve sheath tumor
- Synovial sarcoma, monophasic fibrous type
- Fibrosarcoma
- Extraskeletal myxoid chondrosarcoma
- Malignant fibrous histiocytoma
- Inflammatory fibrosarcoma of the mesentery and retroperitoneum

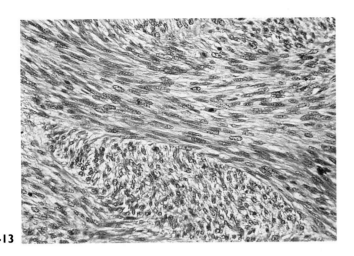

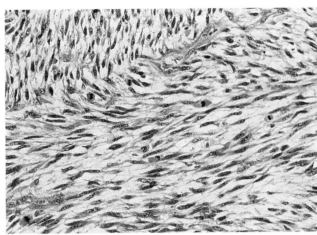

4-13

4-14

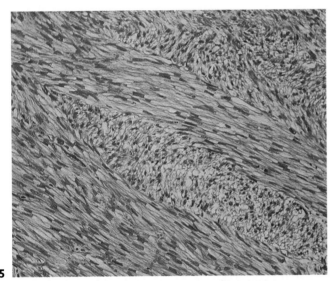

4-15

Figs. 4-13 through 4-15 Well-differentiated leiomyosarcoma: intersecting bundles of smooth muscle fibers in longitudinal and cross-sections. Note blunt-ended nuclei and paranuclear vacuoles in some cases.

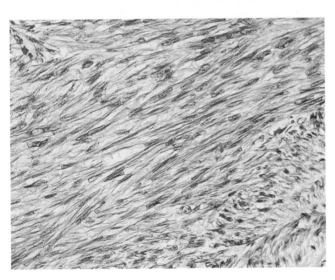

Fig. 4-16 Leiomyosarcoma: Masson trichrome stain showing elongated nuclei and longitudinal myofibrils within the proliferating smooth muscle cells.

Myogenic Tumors

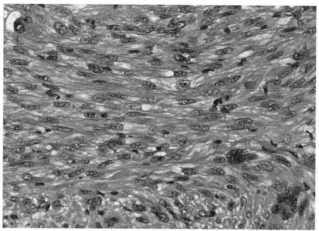
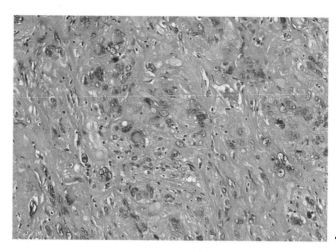

4-17A

4-17

Fig. 4-17 **A,** Leiomyosarcoma demonstrating well-differentiated and **B,** pleomorphic areas similar to malignant fibrous histiocytoma.

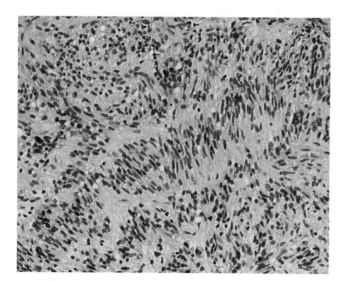
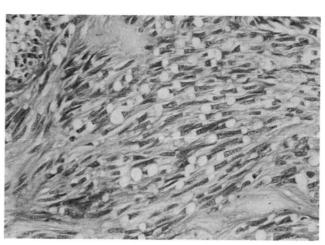

Fig. 4-18 Well-differentiated leiomyosarcoma with prominent palisading.

Fig. 4-19 Well-differentiated leiomyosarcoma with distinct "torch-like" juxtanuclear vacuoles caused by washed-out deposits of glycogen.

Epithelioid Leiomyosarcoma (Malignant Leiomyoblastoma)

Epithelioid smooth muscle tumors have been referred to as leiomyoblastoma and malignant leiomyoblastoma. Those that occur in the soft tissue are extremely rare and usually malignant; they occur most frequently in the mesentery and omentum, and less often in the retroperitoneum. They are distinguished by a prominent round cell proliferation with clear to vacuolated cytoplasm and most likely represent a primitive smooth muscle cell that does not possess all of the attributes of mature smooth muscle, such as intracytoplasmic desmin or glycogen. The criteria to distinguish epithelioid leiomyoma from leiomyosarcoma are not well defined in soft tissue, and the criteria used in the gastrointestinal tract have been used largely by default. These criteria, in essence, state that epithelioid smooth muscle tumors with four or more mitoses per 50 high-power fields (hpf) or greater than 6 cm are malignant, but some epithelioid leiomyosarcomas will undoubtedly be underdiagnosed using these criteria. Epithelioid leiomyosarcomas are capable of metastasizing to regional and distant organs. However, some patients with metastases have survived for long periods, indicating that the prognosis is not uniformly poor.

MICROSCOPIC FEATURES

- Sheets (versus. fascicles) of cells
- Predominantly round cells with scant cytoplasm
- Vacuolated, amphophilic to clear cytoplasm
- Signet ring cells
- Round, central nucleus
- Mild pleomorphism

- Mitoses
- Foci of conventional leiomyosarcoma
- Palisading (rare)
- Myxoid matrix (variable)
- Hyalinization (variable)
- Cystic change (variable)

DIFFERENTIAL DIAGNOSIS

- Poorly differentiated adenocarcinoma
- Round cell liposarcoma

- Signet ring lymphoma
- Myxoid chondrosarcoma

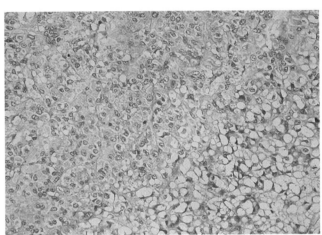

Figs. 4-20 through 4-22 Variants of epithelioid leiomyosarcoma showing round and polygonal cells with abundant cytoplasm, as well as varying degrees of vacuolization and spindling. (Figs. 4-20, 4-21**A**, and 4-21**B** are the same case.)

4-20

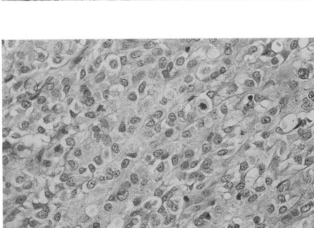

4-21A

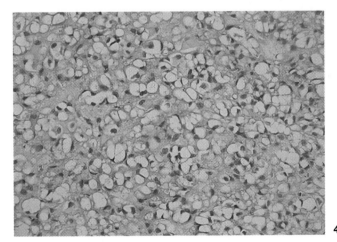

4-21B

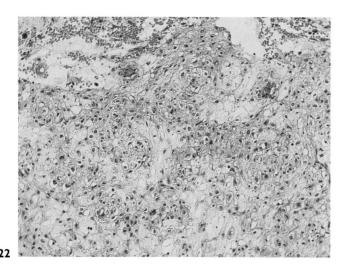

4-22

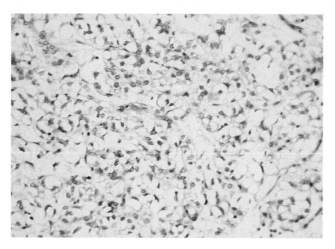

Figs. 4-20 through 4-22—cont'd. For legend, see page 117.

Fig. 4-23 Epithelioid leiomyosarcoma with myxoid change and a prominent vascular pattern simulating myxoid liposarcoma.

STRIATED MUSCLE: BENIGN

Benign Rhabdomyoma

Benign tumors of skeletal muscle are far less common than their malignant counterparts. Rhabdomyomas comprise the overwhelming majority of benign skeletal muscle lesions and consist chiefly of the adult, fetal, and genital types. Whether these are hamartomas or true neoplasms is uncertain, although recent cytogenetic studies on a recurrent case of adult rhabdomyoma showed clonal chromosomal abnor-malities, which supports the concept that these are neoplasms.

Adult Rhabdomyoma

This lesion usually presents as a solitary mass in the head and neck of adults 40 years of age or younger. They are found in males more often than females and usually occur in the soft tissues of the head and neck, especially the cheek, lip, or orbit or upper aerodigestive tract locations such as the pharynx, soft palate, uvula, larynx, and floor of mouth. They are rarely multicentric and rarely recur.

MICROSCOPIC FEATURES

- Well circumscribed
- Round to polygonal cells, closely apposed
- Abundant, deeply eosinophilic, finely granular to vacuolated cytoplasm
- Cytoplasmic cross striations (variable)
- Intracytoplasmic crystalline inclusions (variable)
- Peripheral small nuclei

DIFFERENTIAL DIAGNOSIS

- Granular cell tumor
- Hibernoma
- Paraganglioma
- Reticulohistiocytoma
- Rhabdomyosarcoma

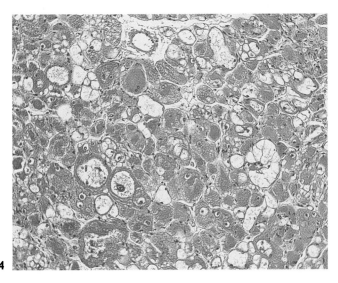

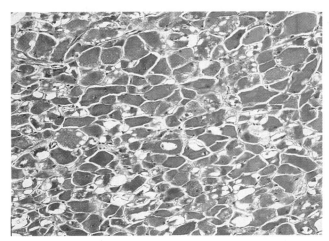

4-24

4-25

Figs. 4-24 and 4-25 Adult rhabdomyomas are composed of deeply eosinophilic, polygonal or rounded cells with small, peripherally placed nuclei. Focal vacuolization, due to washed out deposits of glycogen, is a frequent feature of this tumor. The absence of intracellular fat helps to distinguish the lesion from a hibernoma.

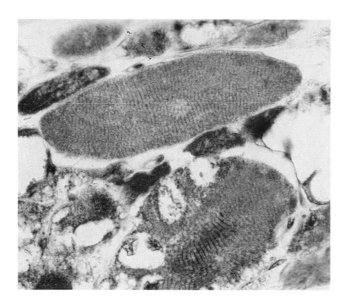

Fig. 4-26 Cells with distinct cross striations in adult rhabdomyoma (PTAH stain).

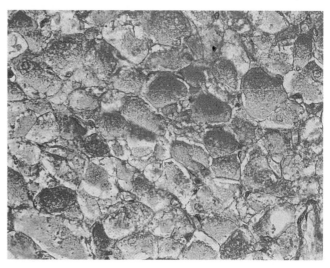

Fig. 4-27 Deposits of intracellular glycogen are a characteristic feature of adult rhabdomyomas. Note glycogen flight, movement of glycogen away from the penetrating fixative.

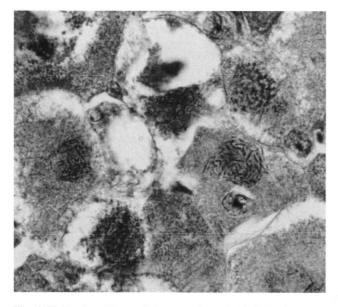

Fig. 4-28 Tangles of intracellular crystals, probably Z-band material (PTAH stain).

Fetal Rhabdomyoma

These lesions are even more rare than adult rhabdomyomas and are presumably hamartomas. Although they have been reported to occur primarily in children younger than 3 years old, they may also occur in adults. They have a proclivity to occur in the subcutis and submucosa of the head and neck, are solitary, and are usually less than 5 cm. Some may be related to neuromuscular hamartoma (benign Triton tumor).

MICROSCOPIC FEATURES

- Well circumscribed
- Undifferentiated spindled to stellate cells
- Scattered immature muscle fibers with a spectrum of maturation (ranging from those similar to 12-week fetal muscle to regenerative appearing adult-like skeletal muscle)
- Cytoplasmic cross striations (variable)
- Variable cellularity
- Prominent myxoid matrix
- Mitoses (rare)

DIFFERENTIAL DIAGNOSIS

- Neuromuscular hamartoma (benign Triton tumor)
- Infantile fibromatosis
- Embryonal rhabdomyosarcoma
- Leiomyosarcoma

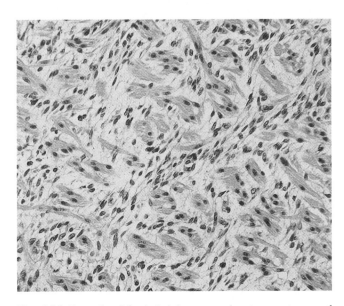

Fig. 4-29 Example of fetal rhabdomyoma showing a mixture of immature, strap-shaped striated muscle cells, undifferentiated spindle cells, and a distinct myxoid matrix.

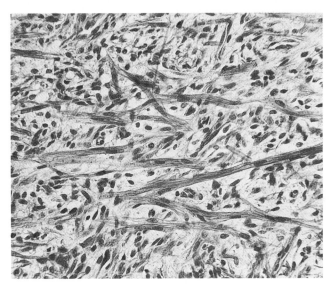

Fig. 4-30 Masson trichrome stain of a fetal rhabdomyoma.

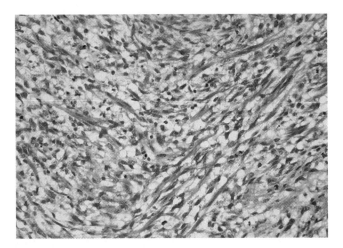

Fig. 4-31 Another example of fetal rhabdomyoma.

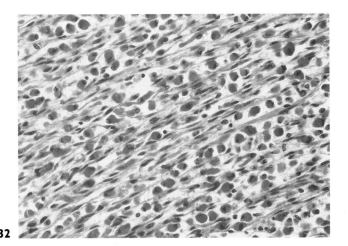

4-32

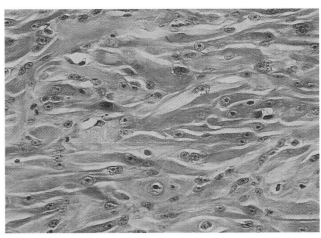

4-33

Figs. 4-32 and 4-33 Examples of the intermediate (or cellular) form of fetal rhabdomyoma

Genital Rhabdomyoma

This lesion usually presents as a vulvar or vaginal polypoid mass in young women and is either asymptomatic or associated with dyspareunia or bleeding. Most are less than 3 cm.

MICROSCOPIC FEATURES

- Poorly circumscribed
- Spectrum of skeletal muscle differentiation (more mature than fetal type)
- Cytoplasmic cross striations
- Mitoses absent
- Abundant collagen

DIFFERENTIAL DIAGNOSIS

- Vaginal polyp
- Botryoid rhabdomyosarcoma

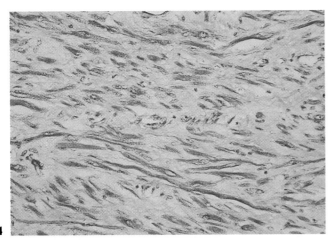

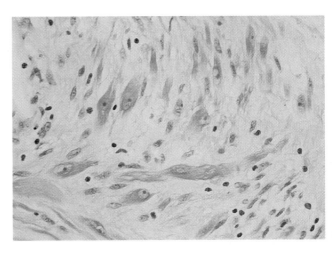

4-34

4-35

Figs. 4-34 and 4-35 Examples of genital rhabdomyoma showing a spectrum of maturation (Fig. 4-34, trichrome stain).

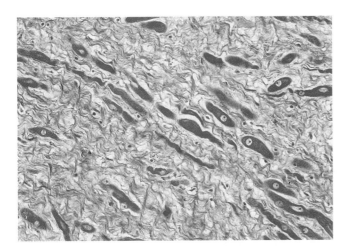

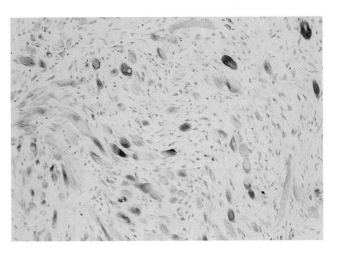

Fig. 4-36 Trichrome stain of vaginal rhabdomyoma demonstrating more advanced rhabdomyoblastic differentiation.

Fig. 4-37 Desmin immunostaining in a vaginal rhabdomyoma.

STRIATED MUSCLE: MALIGNANT

Rhabdomyosarcoma

Rhabdomyosarcoma is the most common sarcoma of children and adolescents. There are basically three types of rhabdomyosarcoma: embryonal, alveolar, and pleomorphic; these categories may overlap histologically. **Embryonal rhabdomyosarcoma** accounts for nearly three fourths of all rhabdomyosarcomas, involves predominantly the paratesticular and the head and neck regions, and occurs primarily in children younger than 15 years old. Two well-recognized variants of embryonal rhabdomyosarcoma are the **botryoid** and **spindle cell** types. The former characteristically occurs along the mucosal surfaces of the genitourinary tract and the head and neck regions and almost exclusively in young children. **Spindle cell rhabdomyosarcoma,** which is extremely rare and simulates fibrosarcoma and leiomyosarcoma, has the best prognosis of all rhabdomyosarcomas. **Alveolar rhabdomyosarcoma** tends to present as a deep-seated mass involving the limbs of adolescents and has a worse prognosis than other rhabdomyosarcomas. **Pleomorphic rhadomyosarcoma** is probably the rarest type of rhabdomyosarcoma; it typically presents in adults older than 45 years of age. Among all types of rhabdomyosarcoma, metastases occur most frequently to lungs, regional lymph nodes, and bone marrow. Bone extension is not uncommon in rhabdomyosarcomas that involve the head and neck and the distal extremities, and meningeal spread may occur in tumors located in the head and neck region. Over the last 30 years, the prognosis for rhabdomyosarcoma has improved considerably as a result of the implementation of standard treatment protocols that uniformly stage patients who are treated with a combination of surgery, radiotherapy, and multiagent chemotherapy.

Embryonal Rhabdomyosarcoma

MICROSCOPIC FEATURES

- Haphazardly arranged and infiltrative
- Fascicles (rare)
- Alternating hypercellular and myxoid hypocellular zones
- Rhabdomyoblasts with eosinophilic, fibrillary cytoplasm:
  1. Fusiform to spindled
  2. "Strap"-shaped or ribbon-like
  3. Round with concentric fibrils
- Cross striations (approximately 60% of cases)

- Undifferentiated, primitive, round to angulated cells
- Round to oval hyperchromatic nuclei
- Mitoses
- Minimal collagen
- Glycogen
- "Spider-web" cells (rare)
- Multinucleated giant cells (rare)
- Myxoid matrix (variable)
- Cartilage or bone (rare)

Spindle Cell Rhabdomyosarcoma

MICROSCOPIC FEATURES

- Fascicular architecture
- Elongated, fusiform rhabdomyoblasts with abundant, deeply eosinophilic, fibrillary cytoplasm

- Elongated, oval nuclei
- Few mitoses
- Collagenous matrix (variable)

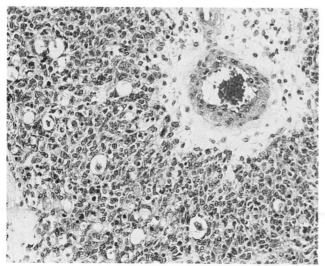

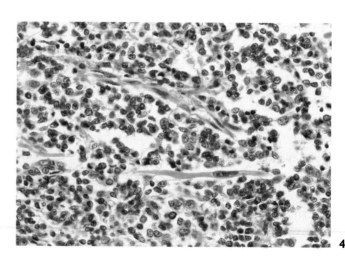

4-38

4-39

Figs. 4-38 and 4-39 Characteristic examples of embryonal rhabdomyosarcoma showing primarily undifferentiated tumor cells and scattered round and strap-shaped rhabdomyoblasts. The clear cells are the result of glycogen storage.

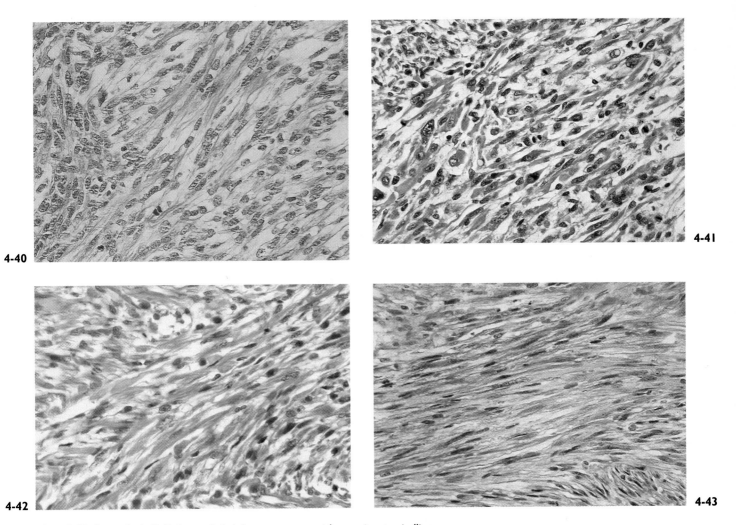

4-40

4-41

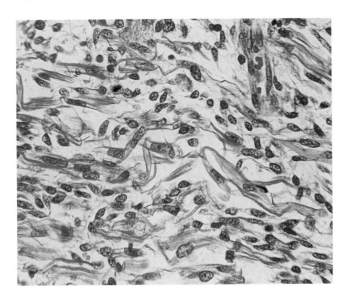

4-42

4-43

Figs. 4-40 through 4-43 Embryonal rhabdomyosarcoma with prominent spindling.

Fig. 4-44 Embryonal rhabdomyosarcoma composed of cells resembling immature fetal myotubules.

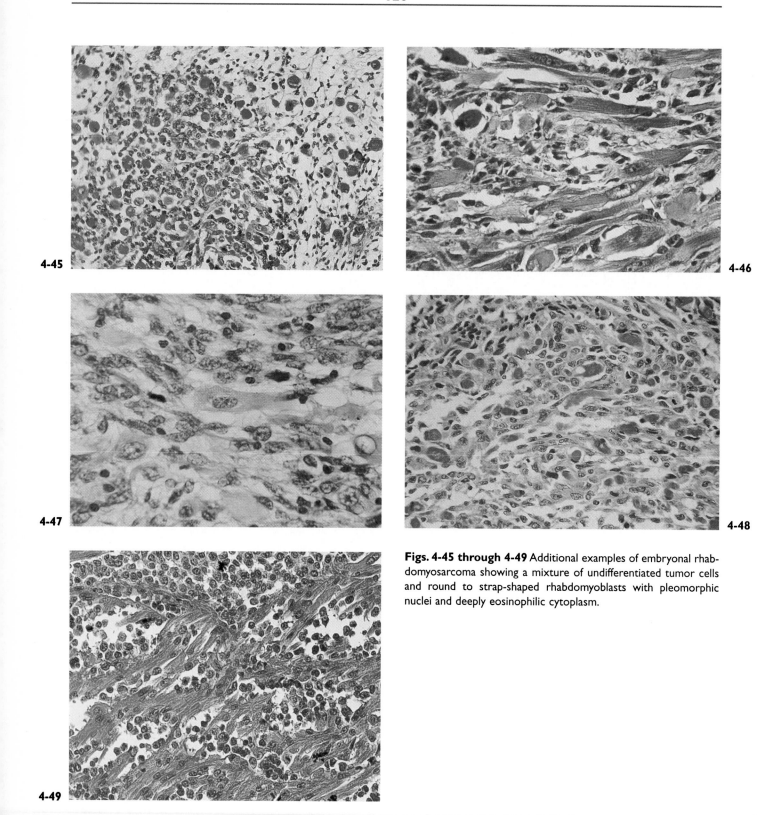

4-45

4-46

4-47

4-48

Figs. 4-45 through 4-49 Additional examples of embryonal rhabdomyosarcoma showing a mixture of undifferentiated tumor cells and round to strap-shaped rhabdomyoblasts with pleomorphic nuclei and deeply eosinophilic cytoplasm.

4-49

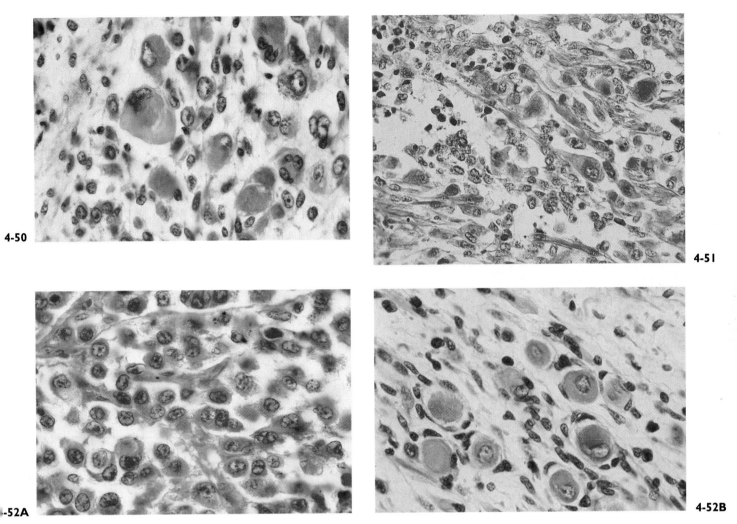

4-50

4-51

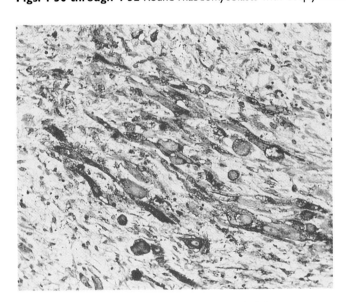

4-52A

4-52B

Figs. 4-50 through 4-52 Round rhabdomyoblasts with deeply eosinophilic cytoplasm at high magnification.

Fig. 4-53 PAS-preparation of embryonal rhabdomyosarcoma showing abundance of intracellular glycogen.

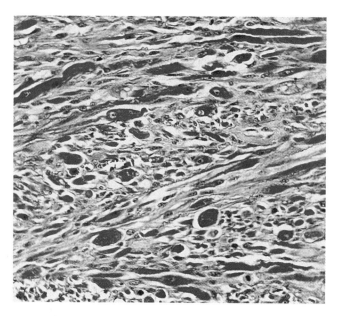

Fig. 4-54 Trichrome stain of embryonal rhabdomyosarcoma showing deep fuchsinophilia of tumor cells.

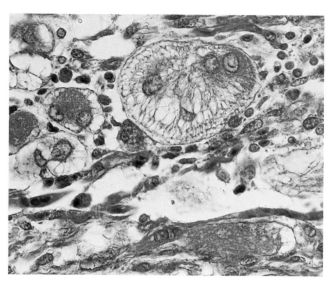

Fig. 4-55 Spider web cells (rhabdomyoblasts rich in glycogen) in embryonal rhabdomyosarcoma (trichrome stain).

Botryoid Rhabdomyosarcoma

MICROSCOPIC FEATURES

- Polypoid growth pattern
- Paucicellular
- Abundant myxoid matrix
- Spindled to rounded rhabdomyoblasts
- Cambium layer (submucosal layer of increased cellularity)
- Cross striations (rare)

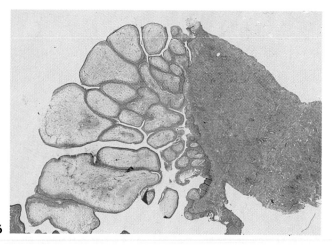

4-56

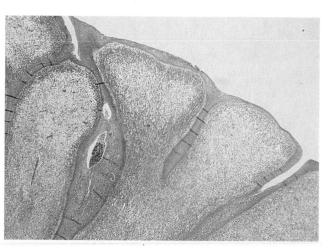

4-57

Figs. 4-56 and 4-57 Low magnification of botryoid rhabdomyosarcoma displaying superficial (intraluminal) myxoid portion and more deeply located cellular area, illustrating the role of tissue pressure in the extent of myxoid change seen in botryoid-type rhabdomyosarcoma.

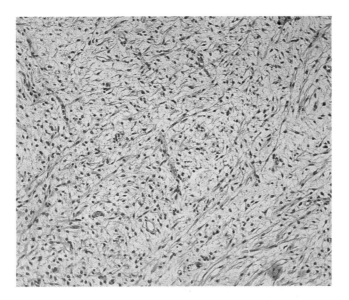

Fig. 4-58 Botryoid rhabdomyosarcoma showing diffuse growth of uniform, undifferentiated, small spindle cells within a myxoid matrix, with and without rhabdomyoblastic differentiation.

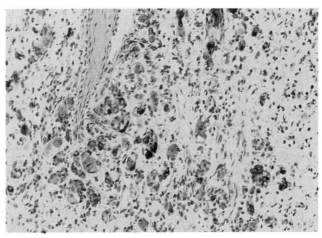

Fig. 4-59 Expression of desmin in botryoid rhabdomyosarcoma.

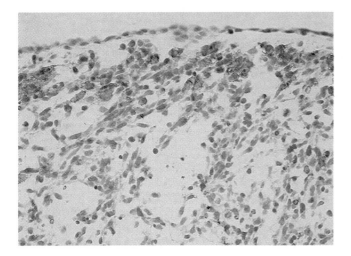

Fig. 4-60 Muscle-specific actin immunostaining in botryoid rhabdomyosarcoma.

Alveolar Rhabdomyosarcoma

MICROSCOPIC FEATURES

- Circumscribed to infiltrative margins
- Prominent, thick, fibrous septa
- Alveolar pattern secondary to loss of cellular cohesion
- Solid, round cell foci
- Acidophilic to clear cytoplasm

- Cross striations (approximately 30% of cases)
- Round to oval to multilobated, hyperchromatic nuclei
- Multinucleated giant cells with a wreathlike nuclear arrangement

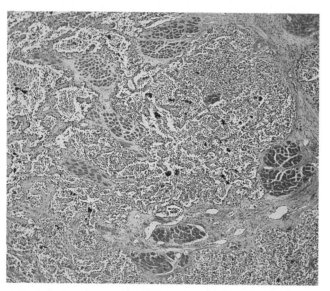

4-61

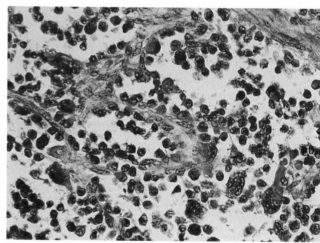

4-62

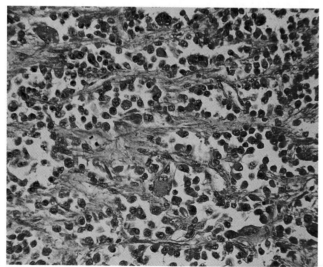

4-63

Figs. 4-61 through 4-69 Typical examples of alveolar rhabdomyosarcoma displaying fibrous septa around irregular "alveolar" spaces, alignment of tumor cells along the septa, and free "floating", partly degenerated tumor cells within the spaces. Isolated or, rarely, small groups of strap-shaped rhabdomyoblasts and multinucleated giant cells also are seen. (Figs. 4-65**A** and 4-65**B** are the same case.)

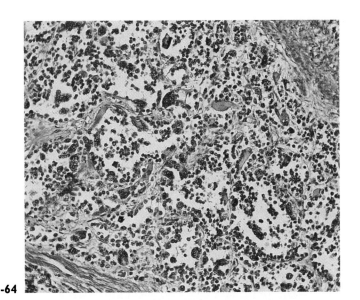

4-64

Figs. 4-61 through 4-69—cont'd. For legend, see opposite page.

(Figs continued on next page.)

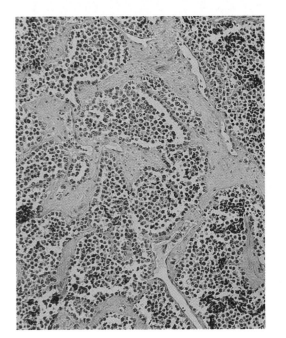

-65A

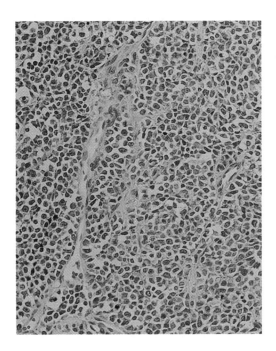

4-65B

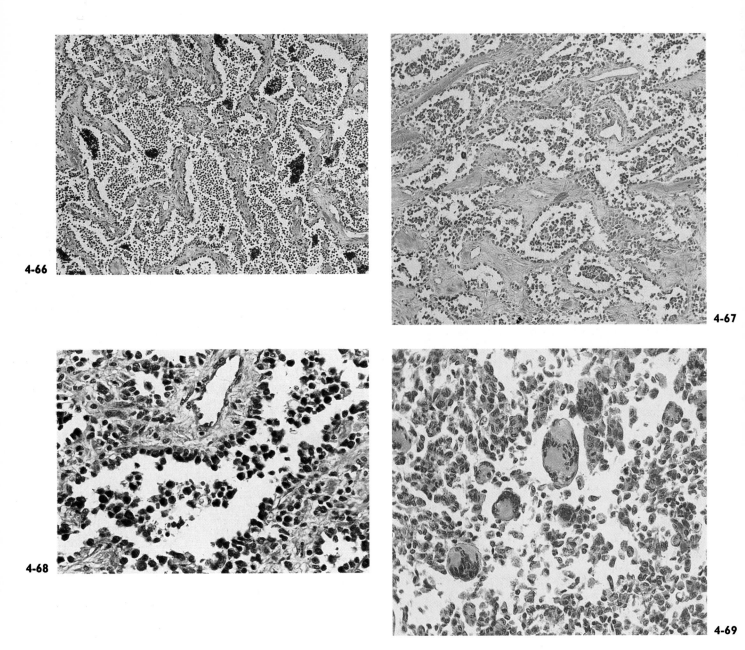

Figs. 4-61 through 4-69—cont'd. For legend, see page 130.

Pleomorphic Rhabdomyosarcoma

MICROSCOPIC FEATURES

- Infiltrative growth pattern
- Disorderly arrangement of cells
- Small, primitive cells
- Large, pleomorphic cells

- Abundant, deeply acidophilic cytoplasm
- Cross striations (extremely rare)
- Minimal collagen

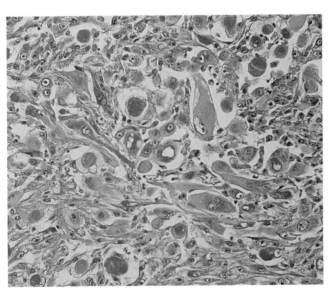

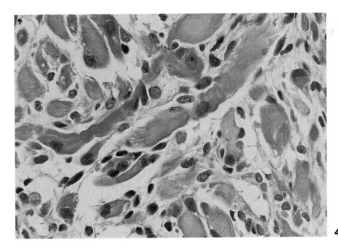

4-70

4-71

Figs. 4-70 and 4-71 Pleomorphic rhabdomyosarcoma composed of variably sized and shaped, eosinophilic tumor cells sometimes associated with small, undifferentiated cells. Cells with cross striations are extremely rare in pleomorphic rhabdomyosarcoma, except for those occurring in small children.

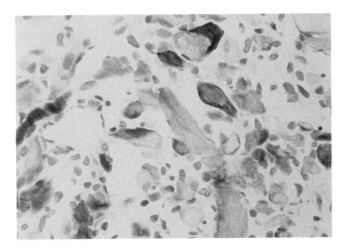

Fig 4-72 Pleomorphic rhabdomyosarcoma, desmin immunostain.

All Rhabdomyosarcomas

DIFFERENTIAL DIAGNOSIS

- Neuroblastoma
- Ewing's sarcoma
- Lymphoma
- Granulocytic sarcoma
- Poorly differentiated angiosarcoma
- Melanoma
- Round cell liposarcoma
- Leiomyosarcoma
- Fibrosarcoma
- Proliferative fasciitis/myositis
- Rhabdoid tumor
- Epithelioid sarcoma
- Alveolar soft part sarcoma
- Malignant Triton tumor
- Ectomesenchymoma
- Malignant mesenchymoma

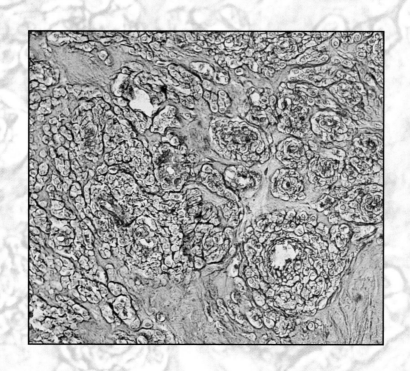

Chapter 5

Vascular Tumors

BENIGN

Hemangioma

Hemangiomas are relatively common soft tissue tumors. There is debate as to whether these are true neoplasms or malformations, but regardless of this controversy they possess limited growth potential. Most hemangiomas are localized growths, but some are diffuse and cover a large area of the body. Some hemangiomas, such as the capillary and intramuscular types, may be diagnosed strictly on histologic grounds, but others, such as the arteriovenous and venous hemangiomas and angiomatoses, require clinical and radiographic correlation to arrive at the correct diagnosis.

Capillary Hemangioma

The most common type of hemangioma, capillary hemangioma, is comprised chiefly of the juvenile and senile ("cherry" angioma) types. It also includes the less common acquired tufted angioma and verrucous hemangioma.

Juvenile hemangioma is the prototype of capillary hemangiomas. It is also commonly known as juvenile hemangioendothelioma or benign hemangioma of infancy. It occurs in fewer than 1% of children and characteristically involves the head and neck region, particularly the periparotid soft tissues. It appears shortly after birth, enlarges rapidly, and not infrequently regresses spontaneously. Lesions that compromise vital structures or cause severe cosmetic problems have been treated with corticosteroids and interferon α-2a. Occasionally, they may be associated with Kasabach-Merritt syndrome.

MICROSCOPIC FEATURES

- Multilobular architecture with arborizing, small vascular channels emanating from a small arteriole
- Plump to flattened endothelial cells
- Variable numbers of pericytes
- Inconspicuous vascular lumina (immature lesions)
- Mitoses
- Interstitial fibrosis with maturation

DIFFERENTIAL DIAGNOSIS

- Cellular angiolipoma
- Kaposi's sarcoma
- Hemangiopericytoma
- Angiosarcoma

Cavernous Hemangioma

This type of hemangioma, which is less common than capillary hemangioma, occurs chiefly in children and involves the upper body. Some may possess a minor capillary component, particularly in the more superficial portions of the lesion. Generally, it is deeper than capillary hemangioma, does not usually regress, and may secondarily destroy neighboring structures. Occasionally, it is associated with other syndromes such as Kasabach-Merritt (thrombocytopenic purpura) and Maffucci's (multiple enchondromas). Radiographically, it is characterized by dilated, tortuous vascular channels and occasionally calcification due to phlebotliths.

A superficial variant of cavernous hemangioma may be associated with multiple hemangiomas of the small intestine (blue rubber bleb nevus syndrome).

MICROSCOPIC FEATURES

- Lobular or diffuse distribution of vessels
- Medium- to large-caliber blood vessels
- Flattened endothelium
- Dystrophic calcification (variable)
- Dystrophic ossification (rare)

DIFFERENTIAL DIAGNOSIS

- Angiomatosis
- Intramuscular lipoma
- Benign mesenchymoma
- Angiosarcoma

Arteriovenous Hemangioma

There are both deep and superficial forms of arteriovenous hemangioma, and radiographic correlation is necessary to distinguish the arterial and venous components. The deep form typically occurs in either the head and neck region or the lower extremities of young patients. It may be asso-ciated with a bruit, clinically significant arterial shunting, and localized hypertrophy as well as require surgical therapy to control symptoms. In contrast the superficial form tends to occur as a solitary submucosal or subcutaneous lesion in adults, has clinically insignificant shunting, and is usually cured with excision.

MICROSCOPIC FEATURES

- Medium- to large-caliber arteries and veins
- Intimal thickening of venous structures
- Capillary and cavernous hemangioma-like areas
- Small capillaries with hyalinized walls and hemosiderin (in superficial zones, simulating Kaposi's sarcoma—variable feature)

DIFFERENTIAL DIAGNOSIS

- Intramuscular lipoma
- Capillary/cavernous hemangioma
- Benign mesenchymoma
- Angiomatosis
- Kaposi's sarcoma

Venous Hemangioma

This type of hemangioma characteristically occurs in adults, is deep seated, and may require venography to be visualized radiographically due to thrombosis.

MICROSCOPIC FEATURES

- Thick-walled blood vessels
- Disorganized muscular wall
- Calcification
- Phleboliths

DIFFERENTIAL DIAGNOSIS
■ See Arteriovenous Hemangioma, p. 139.

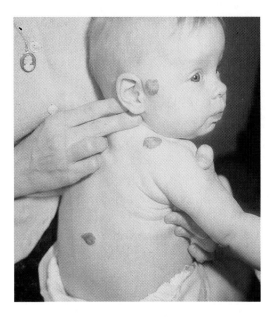

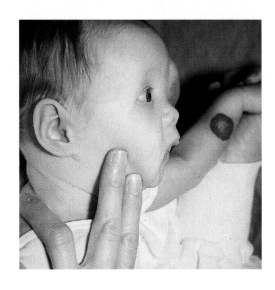

5-2

5-1

Figs. 5-1 and 5-2 Clinical examples of benign hemangioma of infancy (juvenile hemangioma).

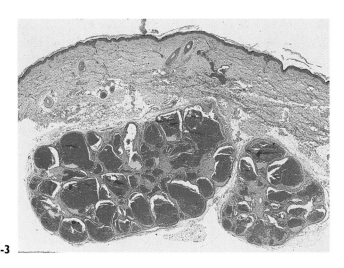

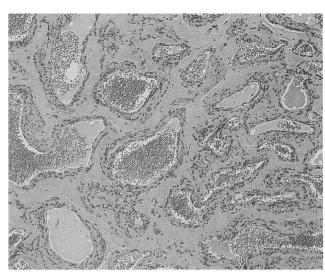

5-3

5-4

Figs. 5-3 through 5-6 Examples of cavernous hemangioma. The thickness of the vessel walls is variable.

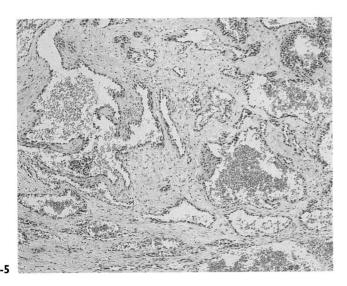

5-5

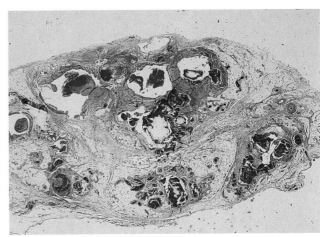

5-6

Figs. 5-3 through 5-6—cont'd. For legend, see opposite page.

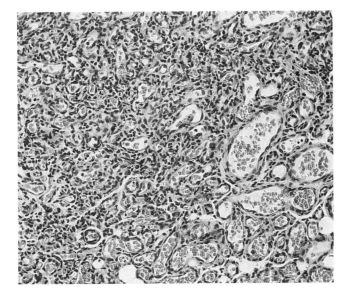

Fig. 5-7 Typical capillary hemangioma with small-caliber vessels.

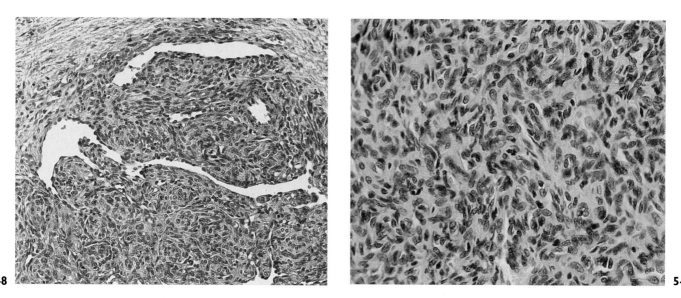

5-8

5-9

Figs. 5-8 and 5-9 Immature capillary hemangiomas in which the lobular architecture is apparent, but the capillary lumina are inconspicuous. Intervascular proliferation of pericytes also contributes to the solid appearance of the lesion.

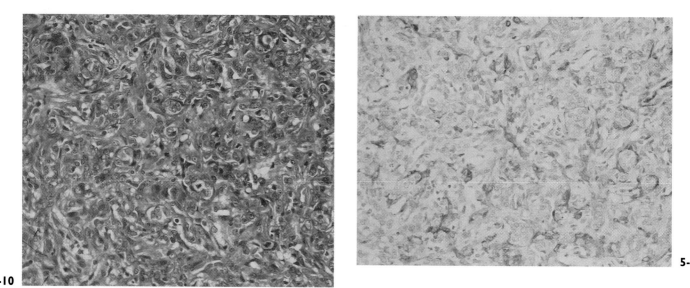

5-10

5-11

Figs. 5-10 and 5-11 Another example of an immature capillary hemangioma that occurred in the thumb of a 15-year-old girl. Occasional small lumina may be seen. This cellular lesion is composed of endothelial cells and pericytes; the latter are highlighted with stains for smooth muscle actin (Fig. 5-11).

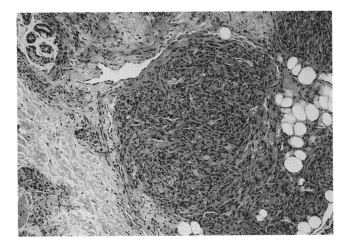

Fig. 5-12 Juvenile hemangioma, capillary type, in a newborn infant, which was clinically associated with Kasabach-Merritt syndrome (giant hemangioma with thrombocytopenic purpura and afibrinogenemia).

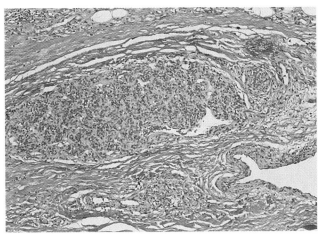

Fig. 5-13 Another immature, lobular capillary hemangioma.

Epithelioid Hemangioma (Angiolymphoid Hyperplasia with Eosinophilia)

As with some of the other hemangiomas, there is controversy about whether this hemangioma is a reactive or neoplastic process. Although evidence suggests that many lesions are reactive, they most likely represent a pathogenetically diverse group.

Epithelioid hemangioma usually presents in the head and neck region of women as solitary or multiple pruritic red lesions during the third through fifth decades of life. Characteristically, the dermis and subcutis are involved, and there is frequently intravascular growth as well. Approximately one third of cases recur after excision.

MICROSCOPIC FEATURES

- Vague circumscription
- Multilobular, frequently with a larger central vessel surround by smaller vessels
- Epithelioid endothelial cells with abundant eosinophilic cytoplasm
- Round to oval nuclei
- Cytoplasmic vacuoles (rudimentary lumina)
- Eosinophils (variable)
- Lymphocytes with germinal centers
- Plasma cells and mast cells (variable)
- Involvement of vessel wall (rare)

DIFFERENTIAL DIAGNOSIS

- Bacillary angiomatosis
- Epithelioid hemangioendothelioma
- Spindle cell hemangioendothelioma
- Epithelioid angiosarcoma

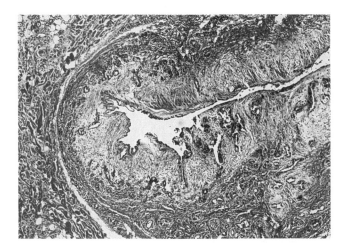

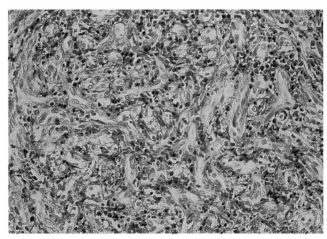

Fig. 5-14 A typical example of epithelioid hemangioma in which a large vessel is seen at the center of the lesion, and smaller vascular channels emanate from the main lumen. Epithelioid endothelial cells can be appreciated even at this magnification. Inflammatory infiltrates, including lymphocytes with germinal centers, may be seen around the periphery of these lesions.

Fig. 5-15 An inflammatory infiltrate with a prominent eosinophilic component often is seen in epithelioid hemangioma. The infiltrate may be so intense that the epithelioid quality of the endothelial cells is obscured.

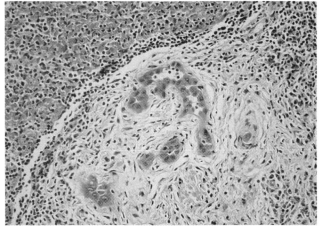

5-16

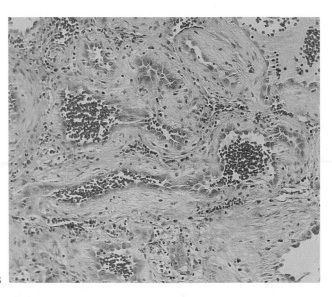

5-17

Figs. 5-16 through 5-18 Additional examples of epithelioid hemangioma in which the epithelioid endothelial cells have abundant eosinophilic cytoplasm.

5-18

Pyogenic Granuloma (Granulation Tissue Type Capillary Hemangioma)

Pyogenic granuloma is essentially a capillary hemangioma that occurs in specific clinical settings. A polypoid growth, it typically presents in the skin or mucosa of the head and neck or the hands. The cutaneous form may be associated with multiple lesions. Some cases occur and recrudesce with pregnancy, whereas other unusual forms may be **intravascular.** Approximately 15% recur; ulceration and satellitosis are not uncommon.

MICROSCOPIC FEATURES

- Well circumscribed
- Polypoid, lobular configuration
- Arborizing capillary channels
- Inflammation (acute and chronic)
- Stromal edema and myxoid change
- Mitoses
- Epithelial collarette
- Epithelial ulceration (variable)
- Fibrosis (variable)

DIFFERENTIAL DIAGNOSIS

- Granulation tissue
- Kaposi's sarcoma
- Angiosarcoma

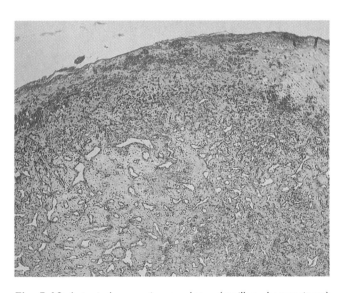

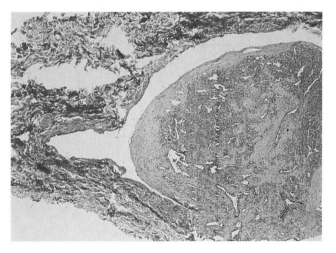

Fig. 5-19 A typical pyogenic granuloma (capillary hemangioma) with numerous thin-walled vascular channels. The stroma is prominent in this case and somewhat myxoid. Note the ulceration of the surface, which is not uncommon in polypoid lesions.

Fig. 5-20 An example of intravascular pyogenic granuloma. There is typically a polypoid intraluminal growth pattern. The lobular architecture characteristic of capillary hemangioma is apparent at low magnification.

Intramuscular Hemangioma

Intramuscular hemangioma usually occurs in young adults younger than 30 years of age; the thigh is the most common location, and the two sexes are equally affected. There are no characteristic presenting symptoms other than a mass effect. Radiographically, these may be hypervascular and occasionally phleboliths are present. Most lesions are of the capillary type, although cavernous and mixed capillary and cavernous forms may also be seen.

MICROSCOPIC FEATURES

- Ill defined and infiltrative
- Capillary-sized vessels
- Cavernous vascular component
- Solid endothelial/pericytic foci with inconspicuous lumina (variable)
- Papillary endothelial tufting (rare)
- Mitoses (rare)
- Perineural growth (rare)
- Adipose tissue (usually secondary to skeletal muscle atrophy—variable)

DIFFERENTIAL DIAGNOSIS

- Intramuscular lipoma
- Benign mesenchymoma
- Angiomatosis
- Hemangiopericytoma
- Angiosarcoma
- Liposarcoma

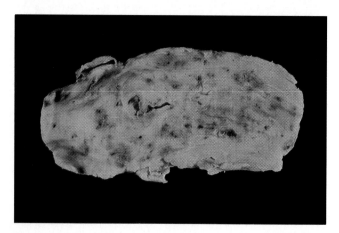

Fig. 5-21 Gross specimen of intramuscular hemangioma. The vascular component may or may not be conspicuous, depending on the caliber of the vessels within the lesion.

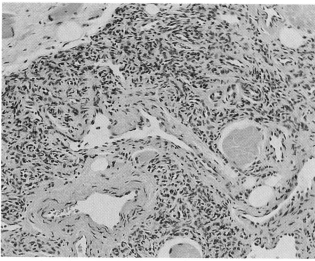

5-22

Figs. 5-22 through 5-27 Examples of intramuscular hemangioma infiltrating skeletal muscle. Fatty overgrowth secondary to muscular atrophy frequently is present. Larger caliber vessels branch into smaller vessels and eventually into capillaries.

(Figs continued on next page.)

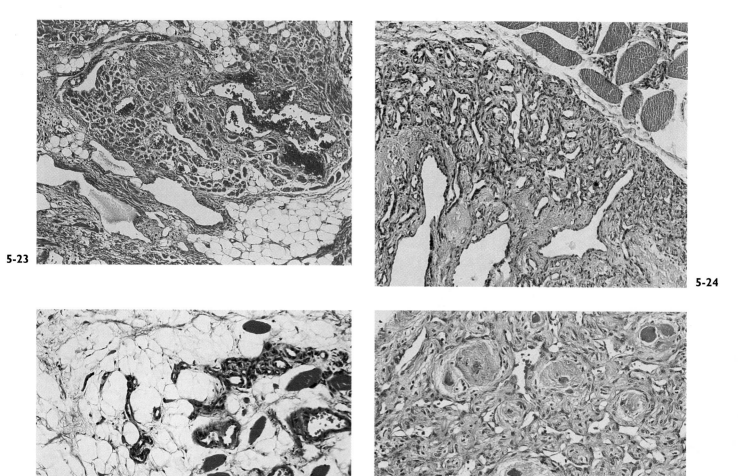

5-23

5-24

5-25

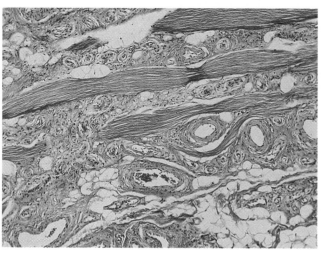

5-26

Figs. 5-22 through 5-27—cont'd. For legend, see opposite page.

5-27

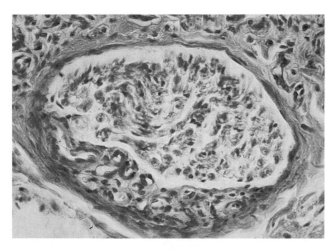

Fig. 5-28 Perineural and intravascular extension are rarely seen in intramuscular hemangioma and should not be misinterpreted as evidence of malignancy or aggressive potential.

5-29

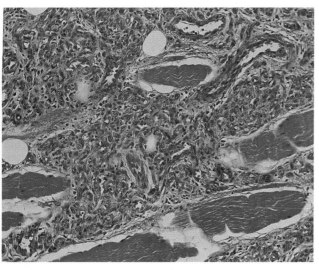

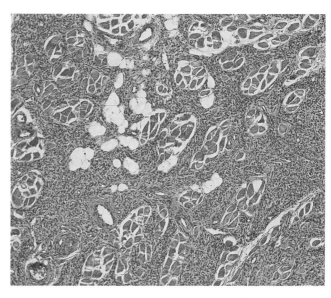

5-30

Figs. 5-29 and 5-30 Additional examples of intramuscular hemangioma; the capillaries are immature in some areas and do not have lumina. Pericytes surrounding the vessels also contribute to the cellularity of the lesion.

Synovial Hemangioma

Synovial hemangioma is extremely rare and can occur within the joint space where it is lined by synovium or along the tendons. The knee joint is the most common location, and the presenting symptoms are usually pain and/or an effusion. These lesions may be either localized or diffuse, and treatment is dictated by the extent of the lesion.

MICROSCOPIC FEATURES

- Localized or diffuse form
- Cavernous hemangioma morphology
- Myxoid or hyalinized stroma
- Hemosiderin deposition
- Inflammation
- Synovial hyperplasia (variable)

Perineural Hemangioma

This lesion is also known as hemangioma of peripheral nerve and is defined as a hemangioma that is confined by the epineurium. The histologic picture is similar to hemangiomas at other sites. These hemangiomas are extraordinarily rare and not unexpectedly are associated with pain and numbness as well as muscular atrophy.

Angiomatosis

This clinicopathologically unique malformation occurs in infants and children and by definition involves a large area of the body such as a limb or visceral organs. The affected structures are enlarged and/or hypertrophic and not infrequently discolored. There may be an associated consumption coagulopathy, as well as repeated local recurrences that contribute to morbidity. Those lesions that impinge on or involve vital structures may lead to the patient's demise.

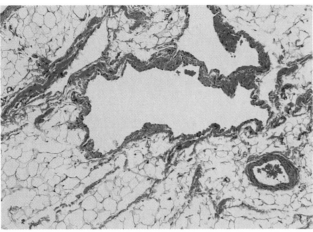

5-31

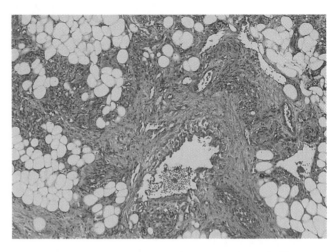

5-32

Figs. 5-31 and 5-32 Cases of angiomatosis diffusely infiltrating adipose tissue. Note the variable caliber of the lesional vessels. The irregular, thin walls of the larger vessels branch into smaller, irregular vessels and capillaries. They are morphologically similar to other deep hemangiomas.

Papillary Endothelial Hyperplasia (Intravascular Vegetant Hemangioendothelioma Of Masson)

Papillary endothelial hyperplasia is an unusual variant of an organizing thrombus that may arise within a blood vessel and occasionally extend into the adjacent soft tissue. Frequently, it is superimposed on an underlying vascular lesion such as a hemangioma. The superficial veins of the head and neck, fingers, or trunk are usually affected; a history of trauma is usually not elicited.

MICROSCOPIC FEATURES

- Usually well defined
- Numerous interanastomosing channels and papillary structures lined by endothelium
- Fibrinous to hyalinized papillary cores/matrix
- Enlarged, hyperchromatic endothelial nuclei
- Fibrosis
- Mitoses (rare)

DIFFERENTIAL DIAGNOSIS

- Hematoma
- Hemangioma
- Angiosarcoma

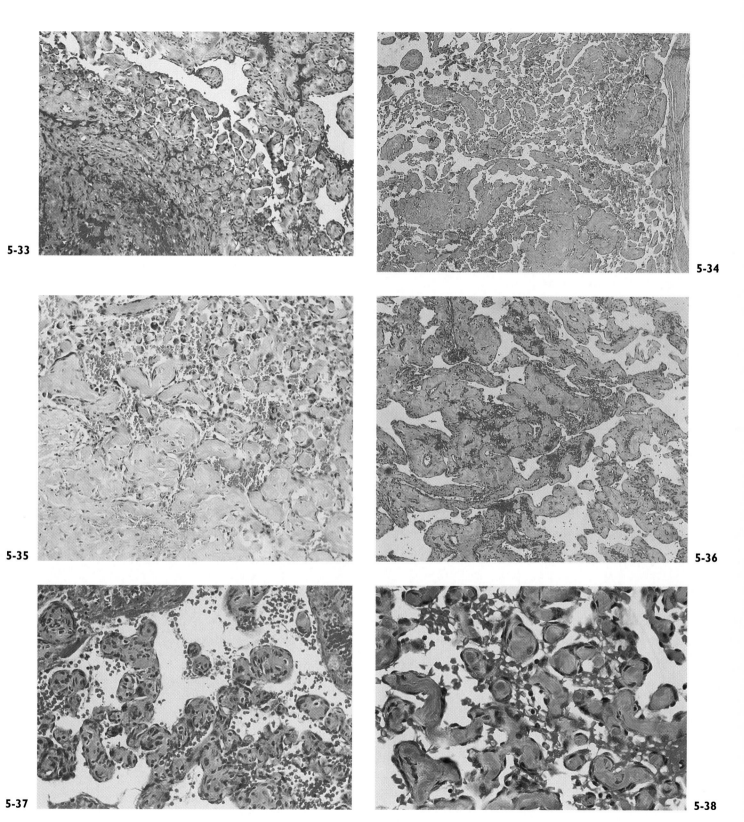

Figs. 5-33 through 5-38 Examples of papillary endothelial hyperplasia. Fibrous papillary cores are lined by hyperchromatic endothelial cells in papillary endothelial hyperplasia. The hyalinized cores of fibrin may coalesce and create the illusion of interanastomosing vascular channels seen in a vascular neoplasm. Tufting, nuclear hyperchromasia, and mild pleomorphism of endothelial cells may all be misinterpreted as evidence of malignancy in papillary endothelial hyperplasia (Fig. 5-38).

Glomus Tumor

There are essentially three types of glomus tumors: (1) the typical or **classic** type, which accounts for 70% of all glomus tumors and occurs predominantly on the fingers; (2) **glomangioma,** which composes 20% of all glomus tumors, occurs primarily on the arm, and accounts for most of the multiple or hereditary examples of glomus tumor; and (3) **glomangiomyoma,** which occurs in the upper and lower extremities and accounts for 10% of glomus tumors. Overall, glomus tumors are relatively rare and have a roughly equal sex distribution (with the exception of the subungual type, which occurs predominantly in women). They occur primarily in the third through fifth decades of life and are often found in sites where normal glomus structures are not found. They usually present as a solitary mass in the dermis or subcutis, are exquisitely painful, and extremely sensitive to cold and tactile stimuli. Roughly 10% of cases recur after conservative local excision. True malignant transformation is extremely rare (see Malignant Glomus Tumor, p. 169).

Classic Glomus Tumor

MICROSCOPIC FEATURES

- Circumscribed (variable)
- Solid sheets or nests of glomoid cells
- Cellular (variable)
- Uniform, round glomus cells with pale to eosinophilic cytoplasm
- Granular cytoplasm (rare)
- Central, round, hyperchromatic nuclei
- Mild nuclear pleomorphism (presumably degenerative—variable)
- Mitoses (rare)

Glomangioma

MICROSCOPIC FEATURES

- Vaguely circumscribed
- Groups or clusters of glomus cells around and in vessel walls
- Cavernous hemangioma-like appearance
- Thrombi (variable)
- Phleboliths (variable)

Glomangiomyoma

MICROSCOPIC FEATURES

- Similar to classic glomus tumor and glomangioma
- Transition between glomus cells and smooth muscle

All Glomus Tumors

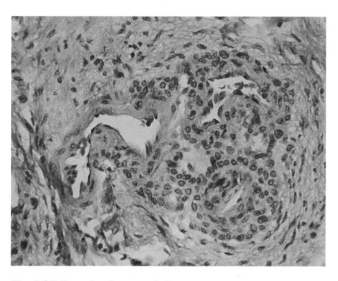

Fig. 5-39 Example of a normal glomus structure.

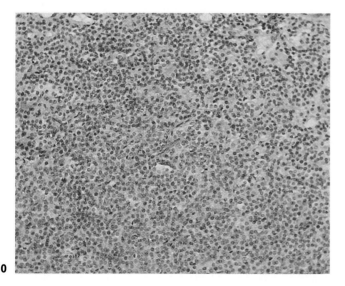

5-40

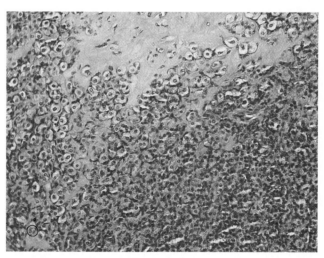

5-41

Figs. 5-40 through 5-42 Glomus tumors with a sheetlike arrangement of uniform round cells. Varying degrees of myxoid change and fibrosis may be seen. Some areas may overlap with glomangioma.

(Figs continued on next page.)

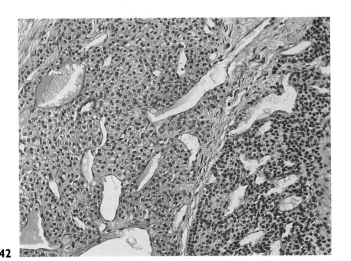

Figs. 5-40 through 5-42—cont'd. For legend, see page 153.

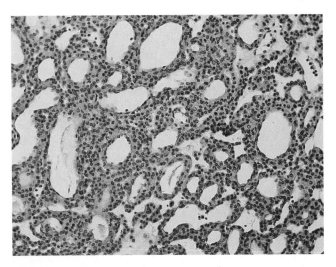

Fig. 5-43 Closely apposed blood vessel walls create a cribriform pattern in some glomangiomas.

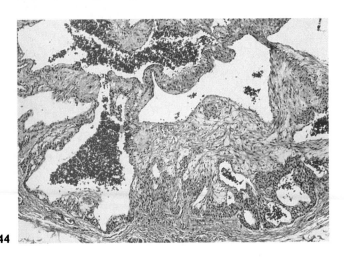

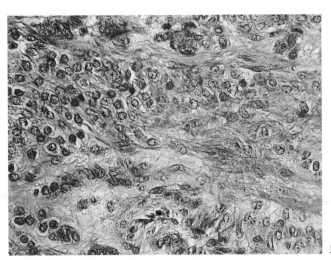

Figs. 5-44 through 5-46 Glomangiomyomas are typified by transitions from glomus cells to smooth muscle (Fig. 5-45, trichrome stain).

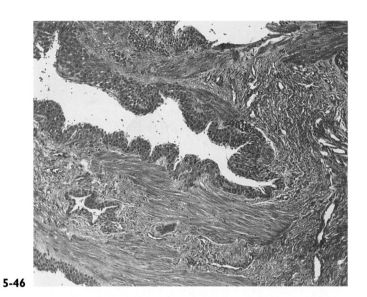

5-46

Figs. 5-44 through 5-46—cont'd. For legend, see opposite page.

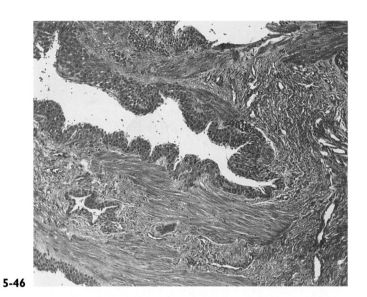

5-46

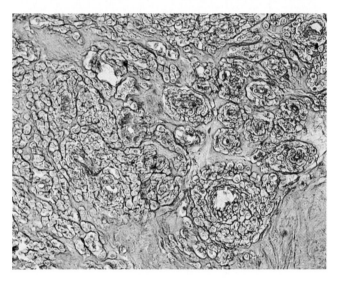

Fig. 5-47 Reticulum-van Gieson stain of a glomus tumor showing investment of individual glomus cells by a basal lamina.

Hemangiopericytoma

Adult Hemangiopericytoma

Excluding the unique infantile variety, hemangiopericytoma occurs almost exclusively in adults. It is usually deeply situated and most frequently involves the thigh, pelvis, and retroperitoneum. Those lesions that occur in the head and neck, such as the orbit, meninges, and nose and paranasal sinuses, share some histologic features of soft tissue hemangiopericytoma, but are best viewed as related but different entities.

Hemangiopericytomas are difficult lesions to recognize because pericytes may display features of endothelial cells, histiocytes, and fibroblasts. Consequently, the diagnosis of hemangiopericytoma is based primarily on architectural rather than cytologic features. Biologic behavior is notoriously difficult to predict. Although a mitotic rate of four or more mitoses per 10 high-power fields (hpf), necrosis, hemorrhage, hypercellularity, and/or nuclear atypia are probably indicative of an aggressive or malignant tumor, histologically benign "outliers" may metastasize 10 to 20 years later. Moreover, location is not predictive of tumor behavior. Metastatic rates range from 10% to 60% and occur most frequently to lungs and bone. Local recurrence is frequently a forerunner of metastases.

MICROSCOPIC FEATURES

- Well circumscribed, with occasional satellite nodules
- Vaguely lobulated
- Numerous, thin-walled, ramifying vessels of variable caliber ("staghorn"-like)
- Single layer of flattened endothelium
- Perivascular hyalinization (variable)
- Large, collapsed vessels at periphery of lesion (near pseudocapsule)
- Intervascular and perivascular proliferation of pericytes
- Relatively uniform pericytes
- Round to oval to slightly angulated nuclei
- Ill-defined cytoplasmic margins
- Sheets or clusters of pericytes
- Small fascicles or storiform foci of pericytes
- Palisading pericytes (rare)
- Reticulin-rich network surrounding endothelium and individual pericytes (variable)
- Myxoid matrix (variable)
- Hyalinized matrix (variable)
- Mitoses (< 4/10 hpf in benign tumors and ≥ 4/10 hpf in malignant tumors)
- Nuclear atypia (malignant tumors)
- Hypercellularity (malignant tumors)
- Necrosis (malignant tumors)
- Hemorrhage (mostly malignant tumors)

DIFFERENTIAL DIAGNOSIS

- Fibrous histiocytoma with hemangiopericytoma-like areas
- Cellular hemangioma
- Glomus tumor
- Juxtaglomerular cell tumor
- Leiomyoma
- Leiomyosarcoma
- Liposarcoma
- Localized fibrous tumor of pleura and peritoneum (fibrous mesothelioma)
- Mesenchymal chondrosarcoma
- Monophasic synovial sarcoma
- Angiosarcoma
- Malignant peripheral nerve sheath tumor
- Malignant fibrous histiocytoma

Infantile Hemangiopericytoma

Unlike the adult hemangiopericytoma, infantile hemangiopericytoma is located in the subcutis and occurs during the first year of life. It is usually a solitary mass that not infrequently is associated with satellite nodules. Despite histologic features that would indicate malignancy in adults, infantile hemangiopericytoma usually has a favorable prognosis; however, in rare cases, it is capable of local recurrences and metastases.

MICROSCOPIC FEATURES

- Multilobular architecture
- Satellite nodules
- Infiltrative (rare)
- Pericytic cells (see adult hemangiopericytoma)
- Occasional intravascular growth
- Mitoses
- Necrosis

DIFFERENTIAL DIAGNOSIS

- Tufted hemangioma
- Infantile myofibroma

- Infantile fibrosarcoma
- Malignant peripheral nerve sheath tumor

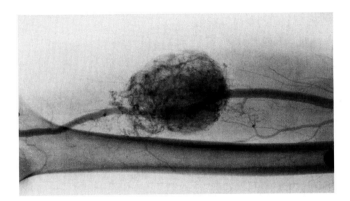

Fig. 5-48 Angiogram of hemangiopericytoma demonstrating extreme vascularity of the lesion.

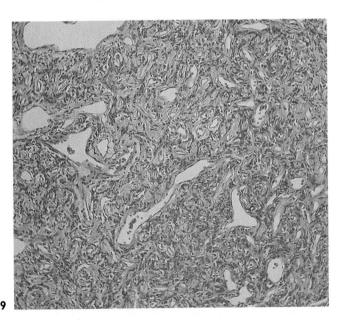

5-49

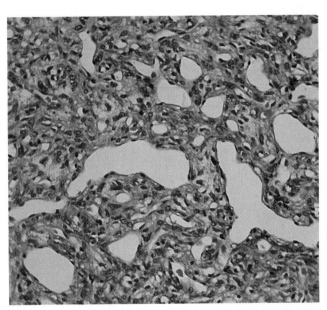

5-50

Figs. 5-49 through 5-53 Typical examples of hemangiopericytoma demonstrating a ramifying or "staghorn" vasculature and a variable degree of cellularity. Hyalinization of the vascular walls is occasionally seen. Large vessels at the periphery of the lesion, especially along the fibrous capsule, are a frequent finding in hemangiopericytomas (Fig. 5-52). Fig. 5-51 is a reticulin preparation.

(Figs continued on next page.)

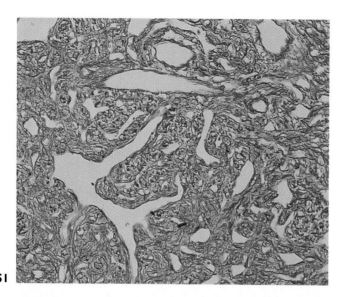

5-51

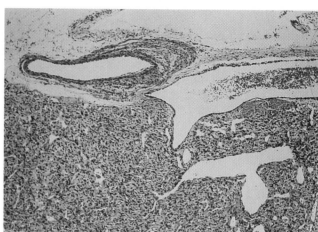

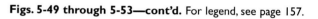

5-52

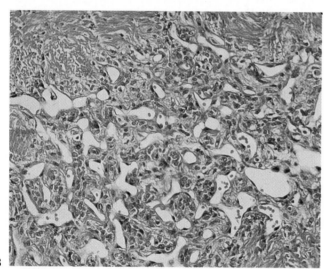

5-53

Figs. 5-49 through 5-53—cont'd. For legend, see page 157.

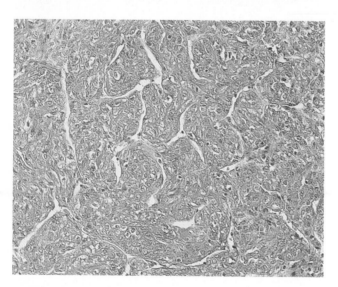

Fig. 5-54 A variable amount of fibrosis or sclerosis may be seen in the matrix of hemangiopericytoma

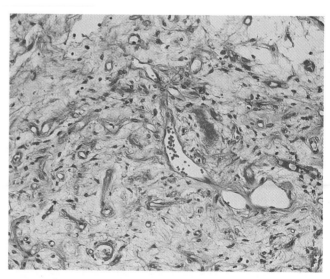

Fig. 5-55 Hemangiopericytoma with a myxoid stroma. This may be either a focal or a pervasive feature in some hemangiopericytomas.

Vascular Tumors

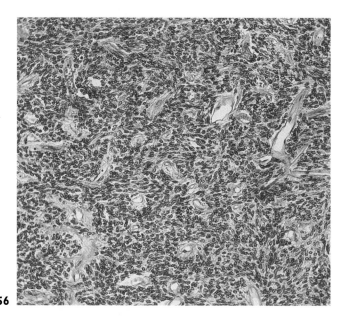
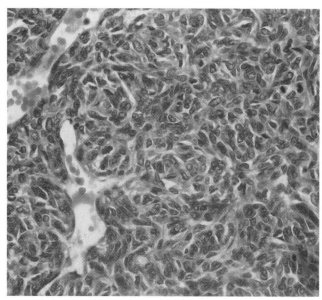

5-56

5-57

Figs. 5-56 and 5-57 Examples of hemangiopericytomas that are probably malignant. In such cases the question of malignancy arises due to cellularity, mitotic rate, pleomorphism, hemorrhage, or necrosis. Some cases may have small, round, primitive cells.

BORDERLINE

Hemangioendothelioma

Spindle Cell Hemangioendothelioma

This extremely low-grade malignant vascular neoplasm tends to occur in the distal extremities of adolescents and young adults. It typically involves the dermis and subcutis and is characterized by a multinodular growth pattern or multiple red lesions in the same vicinity. There are local recurrences in approximately two thirds of cases; metastases rarely, if ever, occur. Some cases of spindle cell hemangioendothelioma have been associated with multiple enchondromas, raising the possibility that this association may be a variant of Maffucci's syndrome.

MICROSCOPIC FEATURES

- Multinodular pattern (or multiple nodules)
- Cavernous hemangioma-like appearance (low magnification)
- Phleboliths
- Primitive but bland spindle cells between gaping vascular channels ("Kaposiform" component)
- Epithelioid endothelial cells with rudimentary (signet ring–like) lumina

DIFFERENTIAL DIAGNOSIS

- Cavernous hemangioma
- Angiosarcoma
- Kaposi's sarcoma

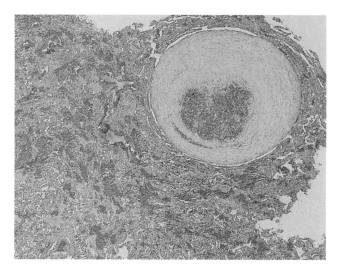

Fig. 5-58 Typical low-power appearance of spindle cell hemangioendothelioma demonstrating cavernous vascular channels and prominent phlebolith.

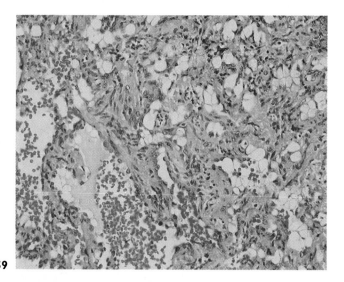

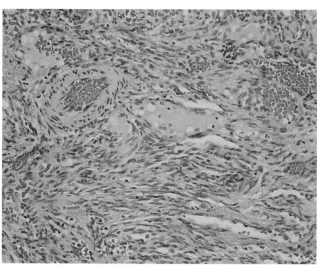

5-59

5-60

Figs. 5-59 and 5-60 Additional examples of spindle cell hemangioendothelioma with cavernous vascular channels, spindle cells simulating Kaposi's sarcoma, epithelioid endothelial cells, and occasional small vascular lumina similar to signet ring cells.

Epithelioid Hemangioendothelioma

Epithelioid hemangioendothelioma of soft tissue is a low-grade malignant vascular neoplasm that usually occurs as a solitary mass in either superficial or deep soft tissues. Multiple lesions in other organs such as lung, liver, and bone are not uncommon. Lesions that occur in soft tissue are frequently associated with a vessel, most commonly a vein. Short-term follow-up (< 5 years) of the soft tissue cases has shown a local recurrence rate of approximately 15%, a metastasis rate of about 30%, and tumor mortality rate in about 15% of cases. These percentages would probably increase with longer follow-up. Metastases are usually to regional lymph nodes, lung, liver, and bone. Histologic features such as atypia and mitoses may suggest more aggressive behavior in some epithelioid hemangioendotheliomas, but they are not entirely predictive.

MICROSCOPIC FEATURES

- Ill-defined margins
- Intravascular growth with perivascular extension
- Abundant chondrohyaline to myxoid matrix
- Cording and nesting of tumor cells
- Epithelioid endothelial cells with eosinophilic, granular to glassy cytoplasm

- Intracellular cytoplasmic lumina (signet ring–like)
- Intraluminal erythrocytes
- Round to oval nuclei that are usually cytologically bland
- Cytologic atypia (variable)
- Mitoses (variable)

DIFFERENTIAL DIAGNOSIS

- Poorly differentiated adenocarcinoma or signet ring adenocarcinoma
- Melanoma
- Epithelioid angiosarcoma

- Epithelioid sarcoma
- Epithelioid malignant schwannoma
- Mesothelioma

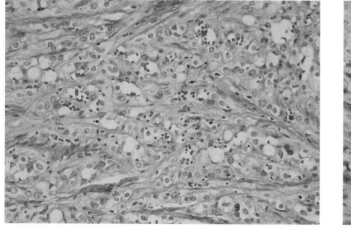

5-61

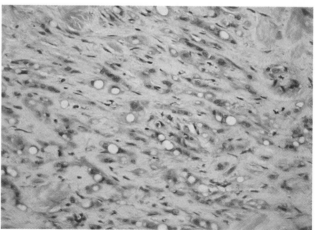

5-62

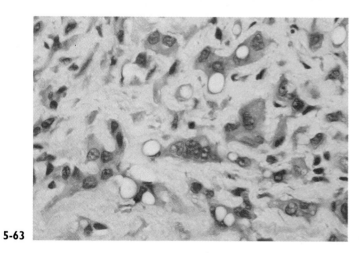

5-63

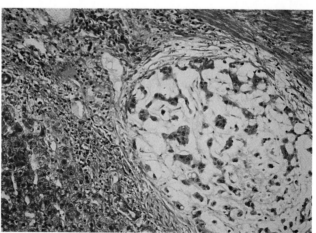

5-64

Figs. 5-61 through 5-64 Nests and cords of endothelial cells with miniature, incipient lumina and a prominent chondrohyaline matrix typify epithelioid hemangioendothelioma (Fig. 5-64, trichrome stain, liver).

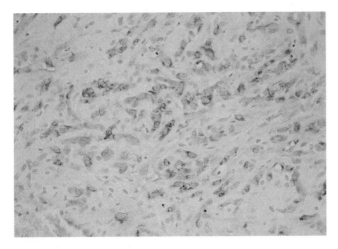

Fig. 5-65 Factor VIII–related antigen in epithelioid hemangioendothelioma.

Malignant Endovascular Papillary Angioendothelioma (Dabska Tumor)

This lesion is an extremely rare and very low-grade variant of angiosarcoma that occurs primarily, but not exclusively, in children and infants. The existence of vascular lesions with hybrid features of epithelioid hemangioendothelioma and Dabska tumor raises the possibility that the two lesions may be interrelated. Although lymph node metastases have been reported in a small percentage of cases, the prognosis remains good with wide local excision.

MICROSCOPIC FEATURES

- Large vascular spaces
- Intraluminal papillary endothelial projections
- Perivascular pseudorosette-like arrangement of endothelial cells on fibrovascular cores
- Cytoplasmic lumina (signet ring–like)
- Intraluminal erythrocytes
- Round to columnar endothelial cells
- Lymphocytes (intraluminal and perivascular)

DIFFERENTIAL DIAGNOSIS

- Lymphangioma
- Epithelioid hemangioendothelioma
- Spindle cell hemangioendothelioma
- Angiosarcoma

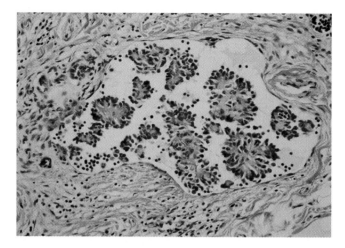

Fig. 5-66 Large vascular channels with intraluminal papillary endothelial proliferations are characteristic of malignant endovascular papillary angioendothelioma.

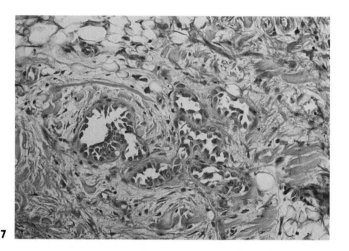

5-67

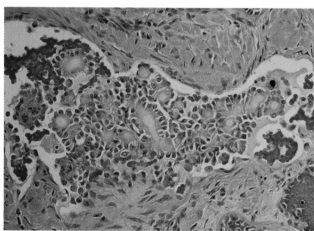

5-68

Figs. 5-67 and 5-68 Additional examples of malignant endovascular papillary angioendothelioma (Dabska tumor) demonstrating intraluminal proliferations of endothelial cells arranged in papillary fronds.

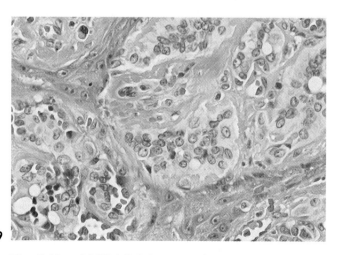

5-69

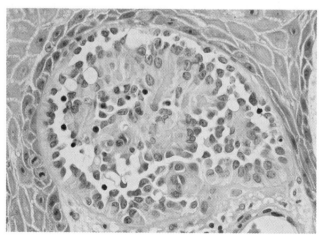

5-70

Figs. 5-69 and 5-70 A Dabska tumor of the abdominal wall in an 11-year-old girl. Some areas overlap with epithelioid hemangioendothelioma. The proliferating endothelial cells stained for vimentin and weakly for CD34 antigen.

MALIGNANT

Angiosarcoma

Angiosarcoma occurs in a variety of clinical settings. The most common scenario is that arising in the skin and subcutis of the head and neck in an elderly individual and unassociated with other predisposing factors such as chronic lymphedema, irradiation, or carcinogenic agents such as Thorotrast, arsenic compounds, or vinyl chloride. Approximately half of the angiosarcomas that occur in the skin and subcutis are multicentric; there is no sexual predilection. Prognosis in these cases is generally poor and largely a function of completeness of excision, which is related to size and multifocality. As with angiosarcomas in other clinical settings, metastases are usually to regional lymph nodes, lung, liver, and spleen.

Malignant vascular neoplasms arising in the setting of chronic lymphedema are considered to be angiosarcomas, and no distinction is made between lymphangiosarcoma and angiosarcoma. Approximately 90% of angiosarcomas associated with chronic lymphedema arise postmastectomy (for carcinoma of the breast). However, less than 0.5% of patients with a mastectomy develop this complication. Lymphedema is usually longstanding, typically of 5 to 10 years' duration. Patients with congenital lymphedema tend to develop a superimposed angiosarcoma at an earlier age than their postmastectomy counterparts, and lymphedema is typically present for 20 years or more. Lymphangiomatosis may be a predisposing or premalignant lesion with respect to (lymph)angiosarcoma.

Angiosarcomas arising within the breast are rare and account for less than 0.1% of all malignant neoplasms in the breast. They typically occur in women who are in their twenties or thirties as a diffusely enlarged breast that may be discolored due to vascular engorgement. Unlike angiosarcomas of skin and subcutaneous adipose tissue, grading is prognostically significant. Most patients expire within 2 years.

Angiosarcoma of the deep soft tissue is rare and information about it is limited. Most cases involve the extremities or trunk, and many are poorly differentiated tumors. In general, these behave as high-grade sarcomas.

MICROSCOPIC FEATURES

- Ill-defined, infiltrative margins
- Multifocal distribution ("skip" lesions)
- Dissecting pattern of invasion between cells, along collagen bundles, and tissue planes
- Irregularly shaped, interanastomosing, sinusoidal-like vascular channels
- Deceptively bland to atypical endothelial lining cells
- Tufted and papillary endothelial proliferations
- Signet ring or primitive vascular lumina
- Epithelioid endothelial cells with granular and/or glassy cytoplasm
- Solid cellular proliferations (poorly differentiated areas)
- Mitoses
- Intraluminal red blood cells
- Lymphocytes (intraluminal and at periphery of lesions)
- Necrosis (variable)

DIFFERENTIAL DIAGNOSIS

- Hemangioma
- Angiomatosis
- Angiolipoma
- Bacillary angiomatosis
- Epithelioid hemangioendothelioma
- Epithelioid sarcoma (with pseudoangiosarcomatous areas)
- Epithelioid mesothelioma
- Poorly differentiated carcinoma
- Poorly differentiated sarcoma

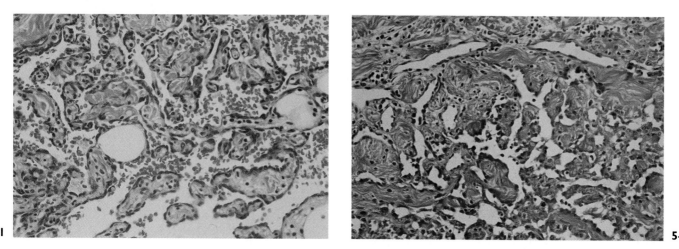

Figs. 5-71 and 5-72 Examples of angiosarcoma involving the subcutis. Note the atypical endothelial cells dissecting through the fat and forming vascular channels. The papillary endothelial tufts are reminiscent of those seen in papillary endothelial hyperplasia.

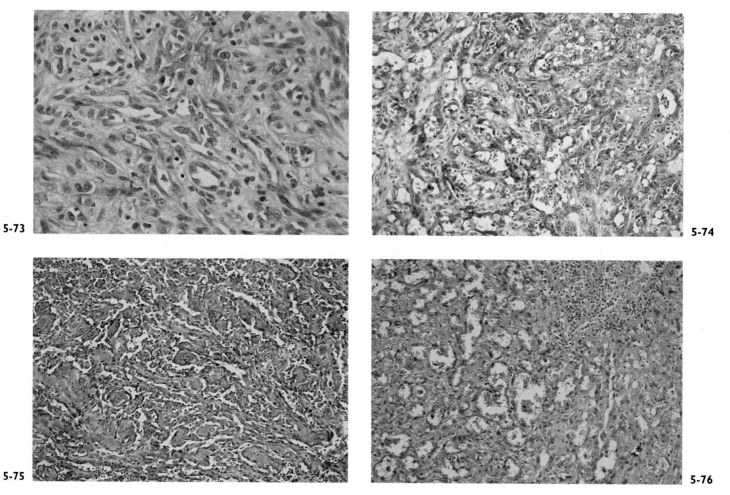

Figs. 5-73 through 5-79 Examples of angiosarcoma showing a wide range of differentiation and nuclear atypia. The lesions display spindle cell areas, mixtures of spindled and epithelioid cells, hemangioma-like foci, and well-differentiated areas with irregular, sinusoidal vascular channels.

(Figs continued on next page.)

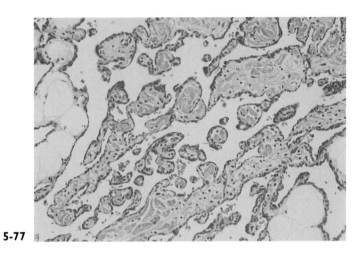

5-77

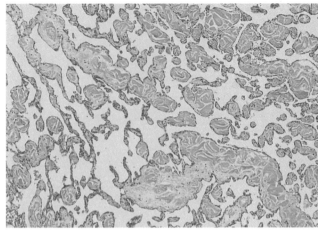

5-78

Figs. 5-73 through 5-79—cont'd. For legend, see page 165.

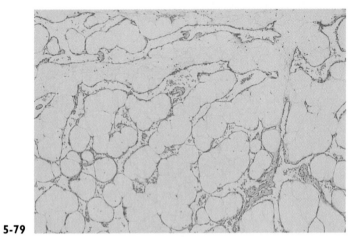

5-79

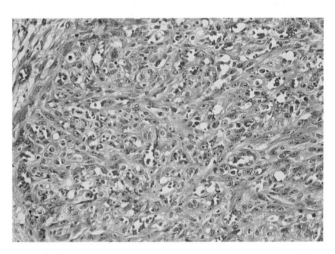

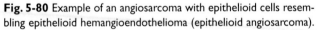

Fig. 5-80 Example of an angiosarcoma with epithelioid cells resembling epithelioid hemangioendothelioma (epithelioid angiosarcoma).

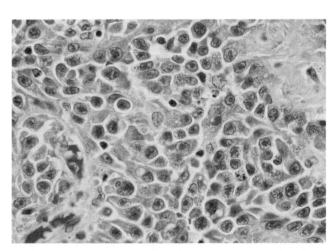

Fig. 5-81 A postmastectomy angiosarcoma in which the endothelial cells become epithelioid to plasmacytoid in appearance, bearing some resemblance to the nodular stage of Kaposi's sarcoma.

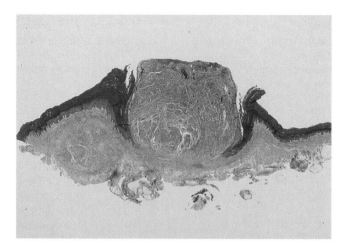

Fig. 5-82 A postmastectomy angiosarcoma with an exophytic and multinodular growth pattern (trichrome stain).

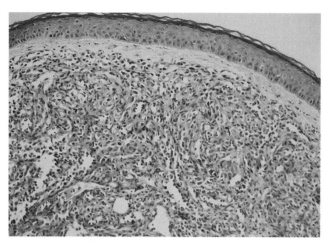

Fig. 5-83 Spindle cell angiosarcoma involving the skin.

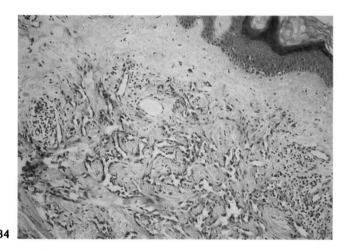

5-84

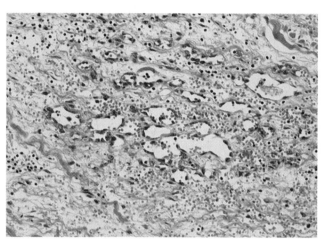

5-85

Figs. 5-84 and 5-85 Subtler areas in the early phases of postmastectomy angiosarcomas involving the skin.

Kaposi's Sarcoma

Kaposi's sarcoma occurs in a variety of clinical settings, but the histologic features of its various settings and stages (plaque, patch, and nodular) are similar.

The classic form of Kaposi's sarcoma is essentially a chronic, slowly progressive disease that waxes and wanes, occurs primarily in older men of Mediterranean or Jewish extraction, and is associated with a second malignancy (usually hematologic) in roughly one third of cases. It has a proclivity to involve the skin of the distal extremities, frequently with lesions of different stages that may coalesce.

Those lesions that occur in association with acquired immune deficiency syndrome (AIDS) are found in a variety of populations including heterosexual and homosexual populations, intravenous drug abusers, and some transfusion recipients. As a rule, the disease course is accelerated in those who develop Kaposi's sarcoma, particularly if there is clinical evidence of involvement of parenchymal organs (such as the lungs, lymph nodes, or gastrointestinal tract) with Kaposi's sarcoma or a superimposed opportunistic infection.

Transplant recipients, another immunosuppressed population, are also at greater risk to develop Kaposi's sarcoma. While the course may be fulminant in this group, they frequently respond to irradiation of the lesion or withdrawal of immunosuppressants.

The lymphadenopathic form of Kaposi's sarcoma is centered in and around lymph nodes and rarely is associated with skin lesions. It frequently affects African children and has an aggressive course.

MICROSCOPIC FEATURES

Patch stage
- Dermal, flat, and ill defined
- Sinusoidal vascular proliferation in lymph nodes
- Dissecting vascular pattern simulating angiosarcoma ("lymphangioma-like" Kaposi's—variable)
- Large, irregular, thin-walled, ectatic vascular channels ("peninsular" sign)
- Proliferation of small capillary-like channels around large, ectatic vessels
- Papillary endothelial tufting ("lymphangioma-like" variant)
- Perivascular lymphocytes and plasma cells
- Hemosiderin (variable)

Plaque stage
- Increased vascular proliferation
- Bland, spindle cells around vessels

- Incipient coalescence of vascular/spindle cell proliferations
- Lymphocytes and plasma cells
- Hemosiderin
- Nodular stage
- Relatively well-defined dermal/subcutaneous nodules
- Curvilinear fascicles
- Uniform, spindled cells
- Slitlike vascular spaces
- Extravasated red blood cells
- Hyaline globules (intracellular and extracellular, PAS +)
- Dilated vascular channels (periphery of lesion)
- Hemosiderin
- Lymphocytes and plasma cells
- Mitoses (rare)
- Pleomorphism (rare)

DIFFERENTIAL DIAGNOSIS

- Decubitus ulcer
- Bacillary angiomatosis
- Hemorrhagic fibrous histiocytoma
- Hemorrhagic nodular fasciitis
- Arteriovenous malformation (superficial portions)
- Nodal angiomatosis
- Castleman's disease
- Hemangioma
- Spindle cell hemangioendothelioma
- Angiosarcoma, well differentiated
- Fibrosarcoma

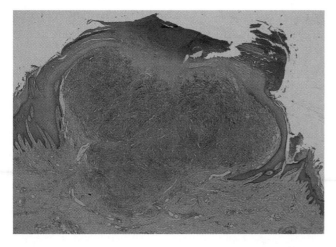

Fig. 5-86 Low-power appearance of Kaposi's sarcoma in the nodular tumor phase. Note the exophytic or polypoid growth pattern.

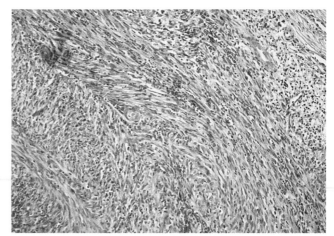

Fig. 5-87 Kaposi's sarcoma showing the characteristic spindle cell pattern with intervening slitlike spaces (slit-cell pattern) containing red blood cells.

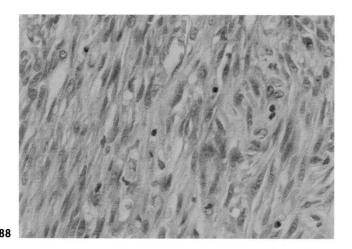

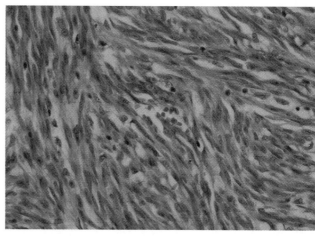

5-88

5-89

5-90

Figs. 5-88 through 5-90 Various examples of Kaposi's sarcoma. Some areas are reminiscent of angiosarcoma, particularly the spindle cell variant, and the morphologic distinction between the two may, on occasion, be difficult. However, the cells tend to be blander than those of angiosarcoma.

Malignant Glomus Tumor

As alluded to earlier, this tumor is extraordinarily rare. Few cases have been reported in the literature. As a rule they are more deeply situated than the usual glomus tumor and tend to involve the underlying skeletal muscle as well as the subcutis. The lower extremities are involved in contrast to the fingers or upper extremities in benign glomus tumors. Cases of metastases have not been reported.

MICROSCOPIC FEATURES

- Fascicular foci resembling fibrosarcoma or leiomyosarcoma
- Areas of benign glomus tumor

DIFFERENTIAL DIAGNOSIS

- Glomus tumor (benign)
- Fibrosarcoma
- Leiomyosarcoma

Vascular Tumors

Malignant Hemangiopericytoma

Many of the clinical and pathologic features of malignant hemangiopericytoma are similar to those of benign hemangiopericytoma. The criteria to distinguish between the two are guidelines and not absolute, although cellularity, nuclear atypia, increased mitotic activity (4 or more/10 hpf), hemorrhage, and necrosis are most commonly used (see Adult Hemangiopericytoma for Discussion, Microscopic Features, and Differential Diagnosis, as well as Figs. 5-56 and 5-57).

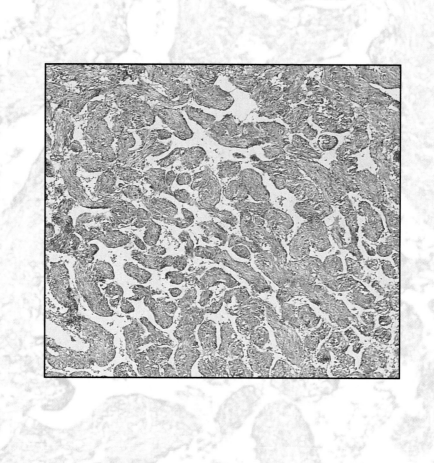

Chapter 6

Lymphatic Tumors

BENIGN

Lymphangioma

Whether lymphangioma is a neoplasm, malformation, hamartoma, or secondary lymphangiectasia is controversial. Most cases are probably developmental defects, but pathogenetic diversity is likely. Lymphangiomas are rare and affect the sexes equally. Over half are congenital, and the majority present before 2 years of age. The overwhelming majority of lymphangiomas involve the head and neck or the axilla, although intra-abdominal soft tissue masses and diffuse or multicentric involvement of viscera may be seen in addition to those associated with hydrops fetalis, Turner's syndrome, and more obscure conditions. **Cystic lymphangiomas** (or **cystic hygromas**) are relatively superficial and circumscribed and composed of large, dilated cystic structures. In contrast, **cavernous lymphangiomas** are more deeply infiltrative within muscle and deep fibrous connective tissue. The former are typically found in the head and neck of infants, as well as the mesentery, omentum, and retroperitoneum; the latter tend to involve the face and mouth. Not infrequently the two morphologic patterns overlap. **Cutaneous lymphangiomas** have a cavernous type of morphology, but the most superficial type, **lymphangioma circumscriptum,** is confined primarily to the superficial papillary dermis. Morbidity is largely a function of location and related to secondary inflammation, rupture, torsion, and infarction. Infiltrative lesions tend to recur, and malignant transformation has rarely been reported in irradiated cases.

MICROSCOPIC FEATURES

- Well circumscribed (cystic type)
- Infiltrative (cavernous type)
- Multicystic, multilobular, or spongiform
- Interanastamosing, thin-walled, ectatic, irregular lymphatic channels
- Irregular thickness of vessel walls
- Disorganized smooth muscle fibers and fibrous connective tissue in vessel walls
- Flat, bland endothelial lining cells
- Epithelioid endothelium (rare)
- Proteinaceous intraluminal fluid containing:
  Lymphocytes
  Lipid droplets
  Red blood cells (variable)
- Lymphoid aggregates in stroma
- Secondary inflammation and fibrosis in stroma

DIFFERENTIAL DIAGNOSIS

- Hemangioma
- Multicystic mesothelioma
- Microcystic adenoma of the pancreas

Lymphangiomatosis

Lymphangiomatosis may involve the bone, soft tissue, and viscera as either a multicentric or diffuse process. Like lymphangioma and angiomatosis, it manifests itself in childhood and has no sex predilection. Those patients with pleural and pulmonary involvement frequently have dyspnea and chylothorax. Approximately 75% of cases are associated with multiple bone lesions. Patients with bone lesions tend to have a better prognosis than those with visceral involvement.

MICROSCOPIC FEATURES

- Ill defined with dissecting margins
- Small and large vascular channels

- Similar to lymphangioma (see Lymphangioma— Microscopic Features)

DIFFERENTIAL DIAGNOSIS

- Lymphangiomatosis with massive osteolysis ("Disappearing bone disease" or "Gorham's disease")

- Angiomatosis
- Well-differentiated angiosarcoma

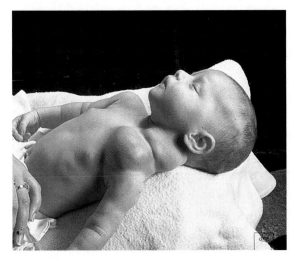

Fig. 6-1 Clinical example of lymphangioma (cystic hygroma) in an infant.

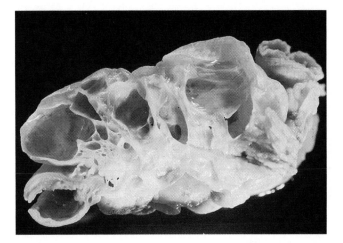

Fig. 6-2 Gross example of a cystic lymphangioma.

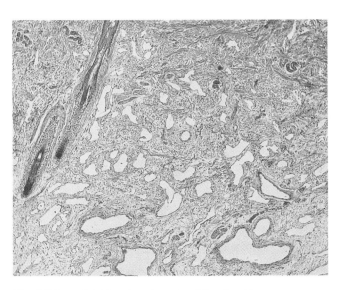

Fig. 6-3 Superficial lymphangioma involving the skin.

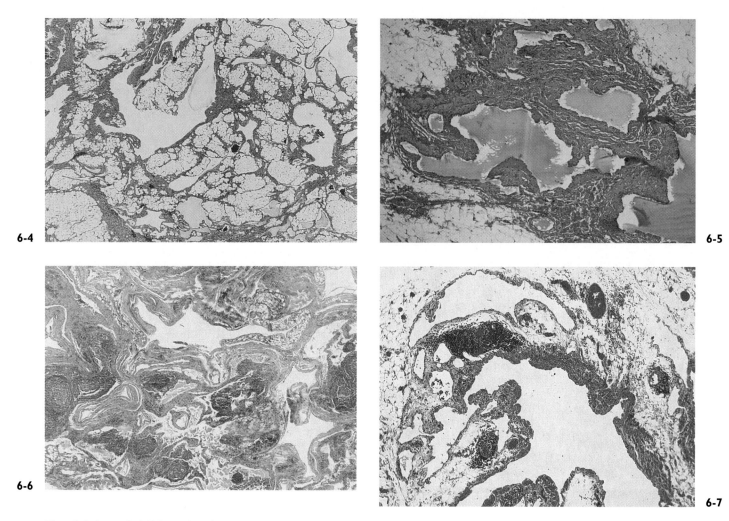

6-4

6-5

6-6

6-7

Figs. 6-4 through 6-7 Examples of cystic lymphangiomas demonstrating variability of the vessel caliber and mural thickness, as well as diffuse infiltration of adipose tissue. Note the intraluminal proteinaceous fluid and scattered lymphoid aggregates.

Lymphangiomyoma and Lymphangiomyomatosis

Both lymphangiomyoma and lymphangiomyomatosis are considered to be hamartomatous lesions; the former represents a localized process, whereas the latter is diffuse. Overlapping clinical and histologic features suggest that it may be related to the tuberous sclerosis complex, although this contention is somewhat controversial. Both lesions consist primarily of a proliferation of smooth muscle in the lungs and thoracic duct, as well as the lymph nodes of the mediastinum and retroperitoneum. Women of reproductive age are afflicted exclusively; they typically present with symptoms of pulmonary involvement such as dyspnea, pneumothorax, hemoptysis, or a chylous pleural effusion secondary to obstruction of the thoracic duct or its branches. Localized lesions have a favorable prognosis, but diffuse lesions do not. Recently, treatment with progestational agents has been beneficial in patients with diffuse disease.

MICROSCOPIC FEATURES

- Angiocentric, short, smooth muscle fascicles
- Disorganization of smooth muscle fascicles
- Smooth muscle fascicles within alveolar septa
- Complex, ramifying vessels of small and large caliber
- Lymphoid aggregates
- Intraluminal proteinaceous fluid (± lymphocytes and lipid droplets)

DIFFERENTIAL DIAGNOSIS

- Lymphangiomatosis
- Benign metastasizing leiomyoma
- Metastatic leiomyosarcoma

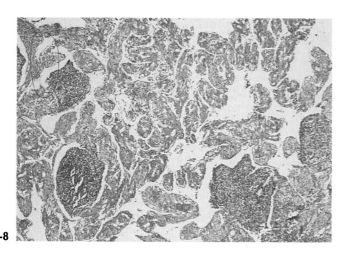

6-8

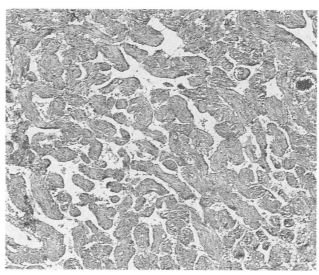

6-9

Figs. 6-8 through 6-11 Various examples of lymphangiomyoma (Fig. 6-8) and lymphangiomyomatosis (Figs. 6-9 through 6-11), with the latter involving the lungs. Note the prominent smooth muscle component and growth along the alveolar septa. Lymphoid aggregates may be prominent.

(Figs continued on next page.)

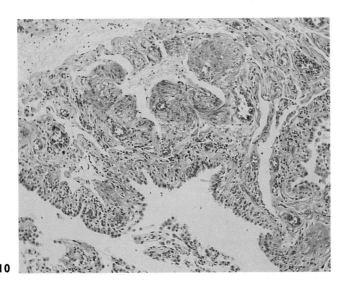

6-10

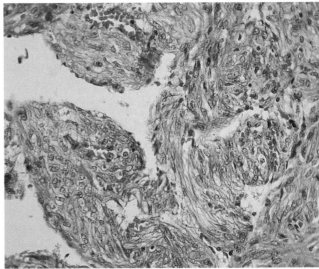

6-11

Figs. 6-8 through 6-11—cont'd. For legend, see page 177.

MALIGNANT

Lymphangiosarcoma

Lymphangiosarcoma arises in chronic lymphedema and is indistinguishable from angiosarcoma.

Most arise postmastectomy and are referred to as Stewart-Treves syndrome (see Angiosarcoma—Discussion, Microscopic Features, and Differential Diagnosis, p. 164).

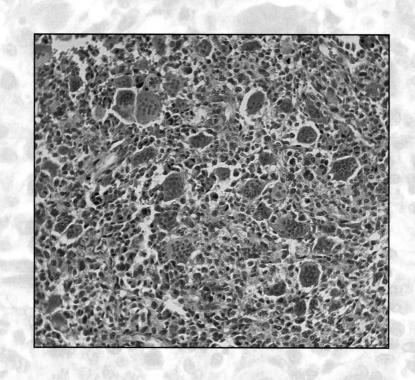

Chapter 7

Synovial Tumors

BENIGN

Tenosynovial Giant Cell Tumor

Whether giant cell tumor of tendon sheath is a reactive proliferation or a benign neoplasm is unclear. In addition, the origin of the proliferating mononuclear stromal cell of both the localized and diffuse forms of giant cell tumor of tendon sheath is controversial. It possesses some histiocytic features, as does one of the two main cell populations of normal synovial cells lining joint spaces, raising the possibility that the two cell populations of normal synovium may have a common progenitor. Despite these unresolved issues, both types of giant cell tumors are well-recognized entities and almost invariably benign in their behavior. There is a histologic continuum between the nodular and diffuse types of tenosynovial giant cell tumor, and distinction between the two, when possible, is based primarily on clinical features.

Localized Type (Nodular Tenosynovitis)

This relatively common lesion occurs preferentially in women in the fourth through sixth decades of life, usually along the extensor or flexor surfaces of the interphalangeal joints of the hand. It is, as a rule, slow growing and fixed to the underlying tendon; approximately 10% of cases are associated with erosion of the underlying bony cortex. The local recurrence rate is 10% to 20% and is most likely due to incomplete excision of multinodular lesions.

MICROSCOPIC FEATURES

- Circumscription
- Vaguely multinodular
- Fibrous capsule
- Attachment to tendon or tendon sheath
- Fibrous septa (variable)
- Mononuclear stromal cells arranged in sheets and nests
- Multinucleated giant cells
- Xanthoma cells
- Hemosiderin
- Chronic inflammation
- Mitoses (variable)
- Intravenous growth (rare)
- Hyalinization (variable)

DIFFERENTIAL DIAGNOSIS

- Fibroma of tendon sheath
- Fibrous histiocytoma
- Chondroma of soft parts
- Foreign body reaction
- Xanthoma of tendon sheath
- Necrobiotic granuloma

Diffuse Type

This lesion could be viewed as a soft tissue variant of pigmented villonodular synovitis of joints. Although several examples of diffuse giant cell tumor of tendon sheath may be associated with bone destruction, this is not a necessary condition. The diffuse giant cell tumor is defined as a poorly circumscribed, infiltrative soft tissue mass that is otherwise histologically similar to localized giant cell tumor. It is rather uncommon and, unlike localized giant cell tumor, tends to occur in a younger patient population and around larger joints such as the knee and ankle. Pain and swelling are characteristic symptoms. These potentially aggressive lesions recur in 40% to 50% of cases, occasionally necessitating radical surgery. Extraordinarily rare cases of metastasizing but benign-appearing diffuse giant cell tumor of soft tissue have been documented.

MICROSCOPIC FEATURES

- Unencapsulated and infiltrative
- Predominance of round mononuclear stromal cells growing in sheets
- High nuclear to cytoplasmic ratio in mononuclear stromal cells

- Multinucleated giant cells
- Xanthoma cells
- Hemosiderin
- Inflammatory cells

DIFFERENTIAL DIAGNOSIS

- Chronic hemarthrosis
- Detritus synovitis
- Xanthoma of tendon sheath
- Localized giant cell tumor of tendon sheath

- Synovial sarcoma
- Alveolar rhabdomyosarcoma
- Inflammatory malignant fibrous histiocytoma
- Giant cell malignant fibrous histiocytoma

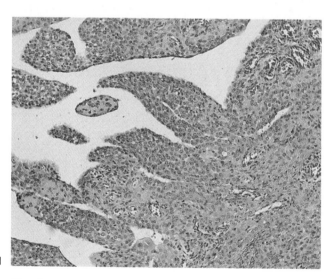 7-1

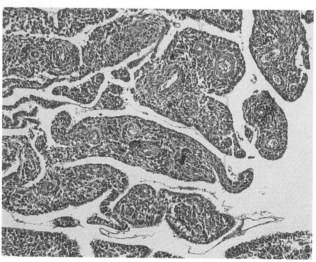 7-2

Figs. 7-1 and 7-2 Examples of giant cell tumor involving the synovium. Classification as localized or early diffuse type in such cases is not always possible.

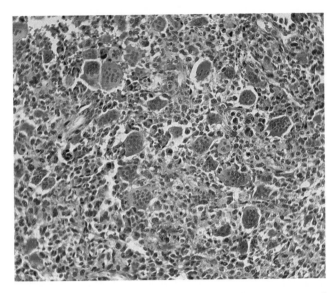

Fig. 7-3 Multinucleated giant cells are a frequent finding in giant cell tumor.

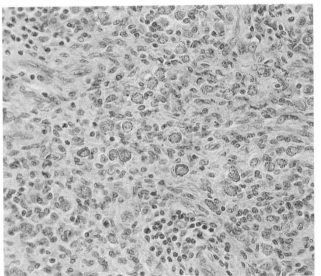

7-4

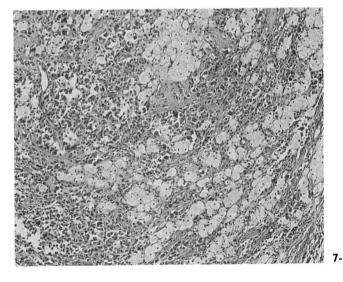

7-5

Figs. 7-4 through 7-6 Examples of giant cell tumor of tendon sheath in which there are varying numbers of macrophages containing hemosiderin, as well as mononuclear stromal cells and background chronic inflammatory cells.

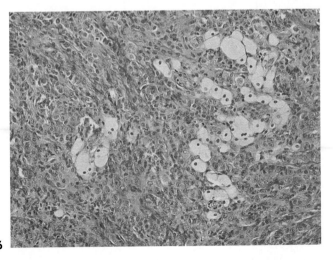

7-6

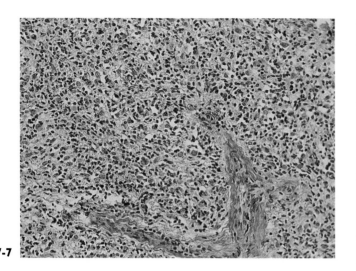

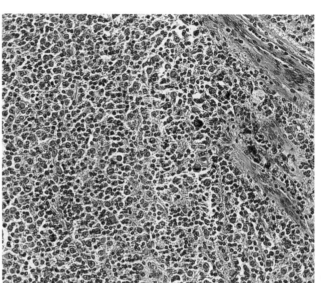

7-7

7-8

Figs. 7-7 and 7-8 Cellular examples of giant cell tumor in which the cell population is more homogeneous than usual and the mononuclear stromal cells predominate. Note focal hemosiderin deposition.

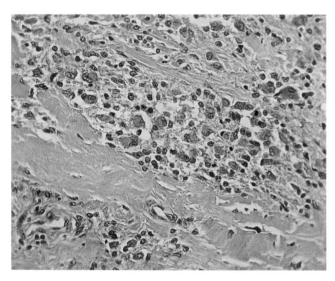

Fig. 7-9 Variable degrees of fibrosis may be seen in addition to plump histiocytes in giant cell tumor of tendon sheath.

MALIGNANT

Malignant Giant Cell Tumor of Tendon Sheath

In these lesions the usual giant cell tumor of tendon sheath is associated with an unequivocal sarcoma such as malignant fibrous histiocytoma, either at its inception or at the time of recurrence. Well-documented examples of this tumor are extremely rare, and generalizations about the few reported cases cannot be made.

MICROSCOPIC FEATURES

- Areas of typical, benign giant cell tumor of tendon sheath
- Prominent and atypical mononuclear cells
- Typical and atyical mitoses
- Hemorrhage
- Necrosis
- Few multinucleated giant cells
- Minimal collagen

DIFFERENTIAL DIAGNOSIS

- See Localized and Diffuse Giant Cell Tumor of Tendon Sheath

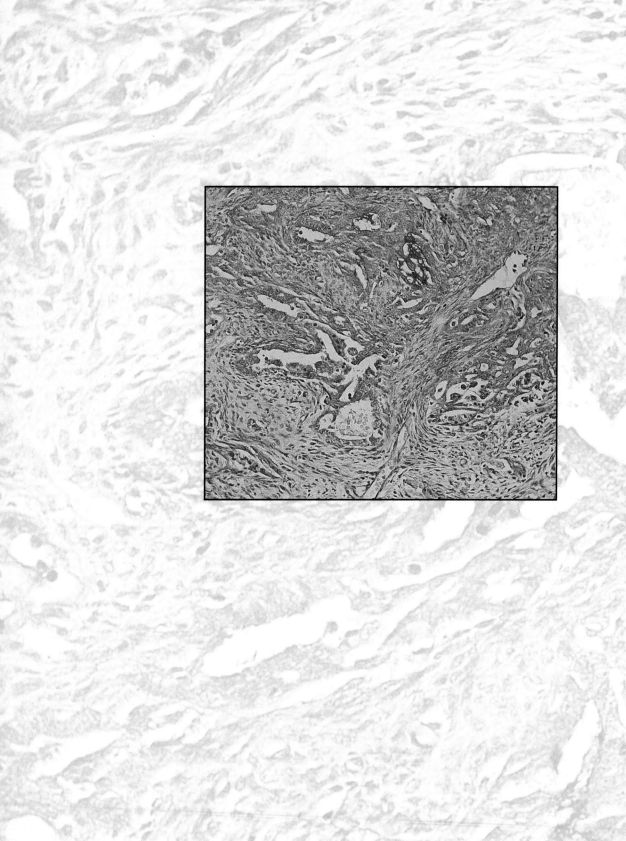

Chapter 8

Synovial Sarcoma

Synovial sarcoma occurs primarily in adolescents and young adults, with males being affected slightly more often than females. It is almost invariably a deep-seated mass near a large joint, especially the knee, or other periarticular tendinous structures or bursa. Characteristically, it is a slowly growing mass that is associated with pain more frequently than other sarcomas. Approximately 20% are associated with bone involvement and 30% are calcified. Although the survival rate has slightly improved with the introduction of multiagent chemotherapy, late recurrences and metastases are not uncommon; metastases are most frequently to the lungs, followed by the lymph nodes and bone marrow. Reported favorable prognostic factors are tumor size less than or equal to 5 cm, a patient age of 15 years or younger, a diploid tumor cell population, a low mitotic rate, and extensive tumor calcification. There is controversy over the prognostic significance of histologic subclassification, although there is general agreement that poorly differentiated tumors (which tend to have a higher mitotic rate) have a worse prognosis than other types.

Four main histologic subtypes of synovial sarcoma merge with each other histologically: the **biphasic, monophasic fibrous, epithelial predominant,** and **poorly differentiated** types.

MICROSCOPIC FEATURES

- Well circumscribed, with a pseudocapsule
- Vaguely multinodular architecture
- Hemorrhagic or mucinous cysts
- Epithelial cells: columnar, cuboidal, to flattened
- Squamous metaplasia (rare)
- Papillary epithelial projections
- Fibrosarcoma-like fascicles and whorls of spindled cells
- Uniform round to spindled cells with a high nuclear to cytoplasmic ratio
- Small round cells similar to Ewing's sarcoma (rare)
- Mitoses (especially in poorly differentiated lesions)
- Mast cells
- Focal hemangiopericytoma-like vascular pattern
- Fibrous bands or matrix
- Calcification
- Myxoid change (variable)
- Chondroid or osseous foci (rare)
- Pseudoalveolar foci (loss of cellular cohesion—rare)
- Nuclear palisading (rare)
- Pseudorosettes (rare)

DIFFERENTIAL DIAGNOSIS

- Hemangiopericytoma
- Fibrosarcoma
- Malignant peripheral nerve sheath tumor
- Ewing's sarcoma
- Peripheral neuroepithelioma
- Epithelioid sarcoma
- Clear cell sarcoma
- Mesothelioma
- Carcinosarcoma
- Carcinoma, especially of adnexal origin

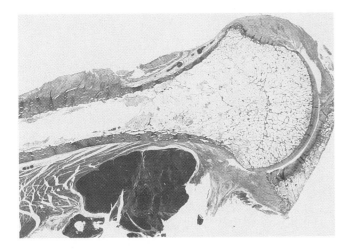

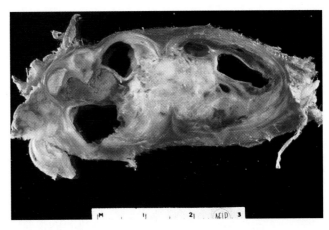

Fig. 8-2 Prominent cyst formation in a synovial sarcoma.

Fig. 8-1 Synovial sarcoma abutting on bone.

8-3

8-4

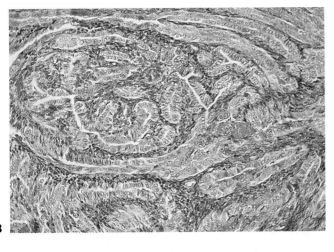

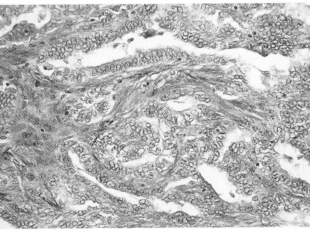

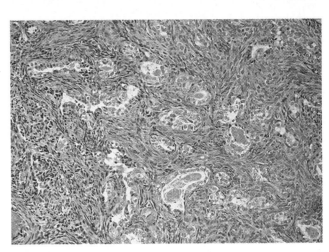

8-5

8-6

Figs. 8-3 through 8-6 Typical examples of biphasic synovial sarcoma with epithelial and spindle cell/fibrous components.

Synovial Sarcoma

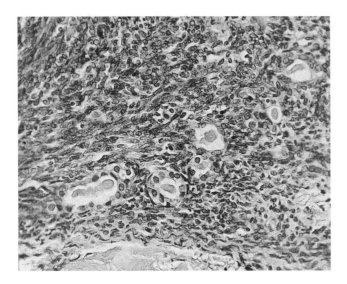

Fig. 8-7 A biphasic synovial sarcoma with small mucin-filled acini.

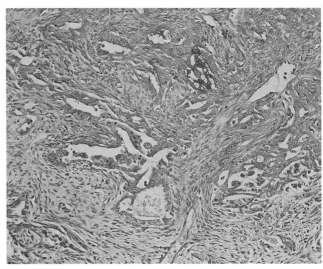

Fig. 8-8 Biphasic synovial sarcoma showing focal myxoid changes in the spindle cell component (PAS-preparation).

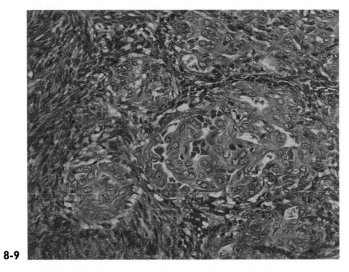

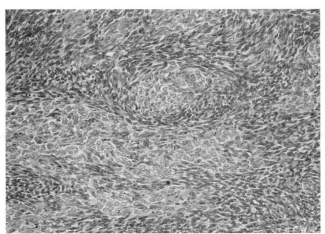

8-9

8-10

Figs. 8-9 and 8-10 Nests of squamous epithelial cells in biphasic synovial sarcoma.

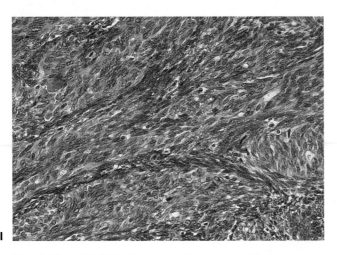

8-11

8-12

Figs. 8-11 and 8-12 Biphasic synovial sarcomas with less conspicuous epithelial components.

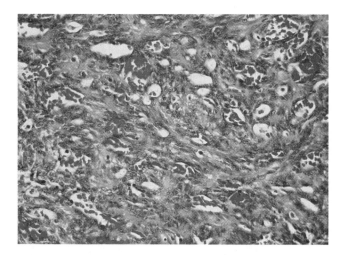

Fig. 8-13 A biphasic synovial sarcoma with hemorrhage resembling an angiosarcoma.

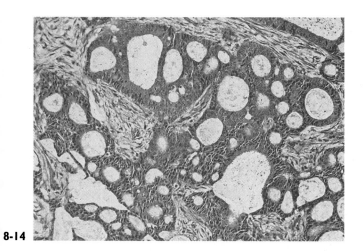

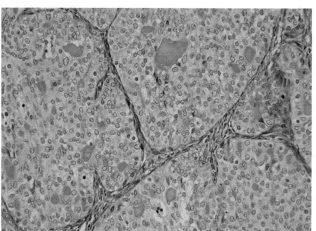

Figs. 8-14 and 8-15 Examples of epithelial predominant synovial sarcoma.

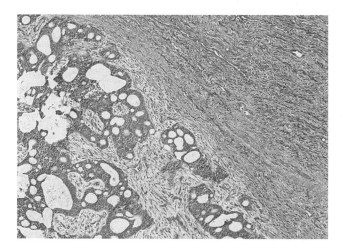

Fig. 8-16 Biphasic synovial sarcoma displaying both epithelial and spindle cell features.

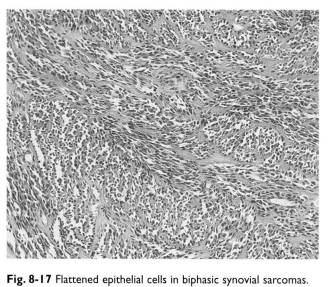

8-17

Fig. 8-17 Flattened epithelial cells in biphasic synovial sarcomas.

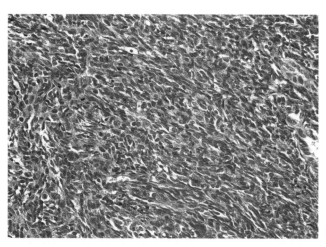

8-18

Fig. 8-18 Poorly differentiated synovial sarcoma exhibiting both epithelial and spindle cell features.

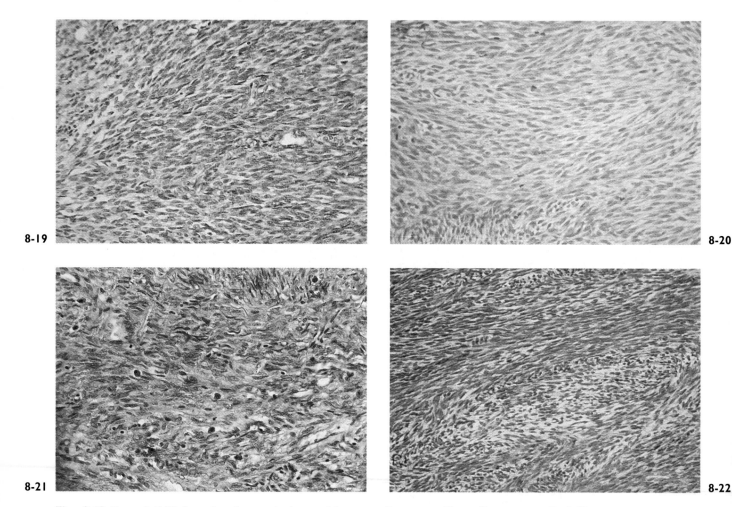

8-19

8-20

8-21

8-22

Figs. 8-19 through 8-22 Examples of monophasic synovial sarcoma, fibrous type. Mast cells are seen in Fig. 8-21.

Synovial Sarcoma

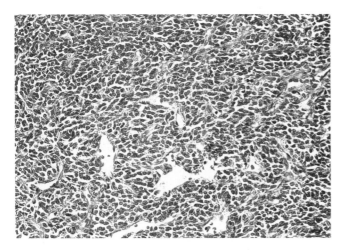

Fig. 8-23 Monophasic fibrous synovial sarcoma with a primitive round cell pattern and dilated vascular spaces

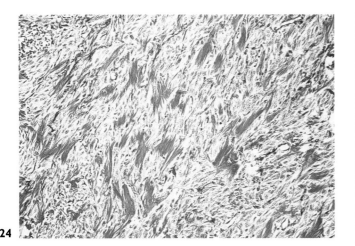

8-24

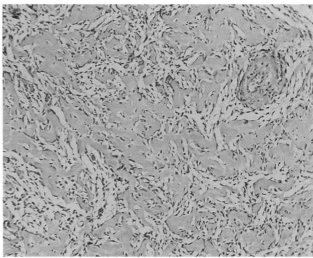

8-25

Figs. 8-24 through 8-26 Various patterns of fibrosis in monophasic fibrous synovial sarcoma.

8-26

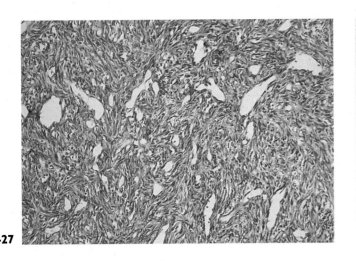

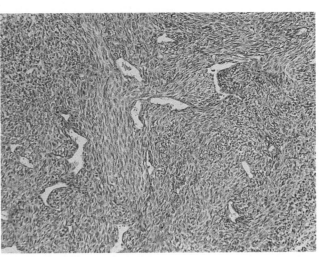

8-27

8-28

Figs. 8-27 and 8-28 Examples of synovial sarcoma displaying a hemangiopericytoma-like vascular pattern.

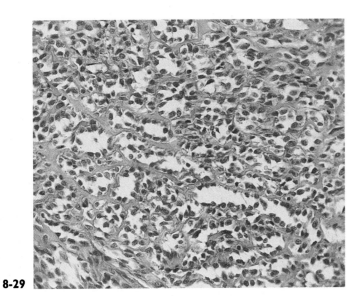

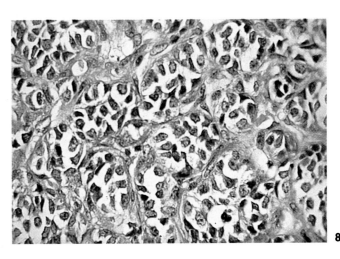

8-29

8-30

Figs. 8-29 and 8-30 Pseudoalveolar patterns present in synovial sarcoma.

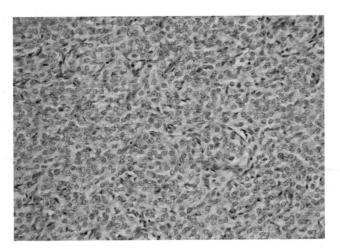

Fig. 8-31 A primitive round cell population reminiscent of Ewing's sarcoma in a monophasic synovial sarcoma.

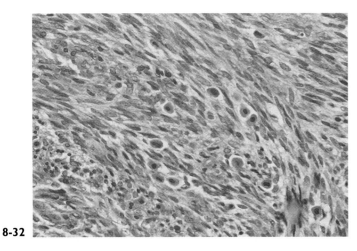

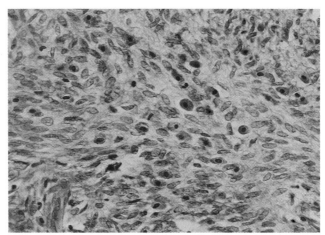

8-32

8-33

Figs. 8-32 and 8-33 Prominent mast cell infiltrates in synovial sarcoma.

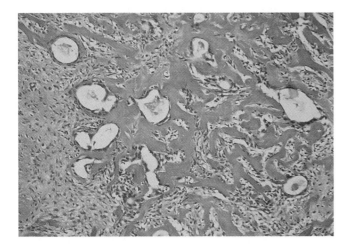

Fig. 8-34 Marked sclerosis in biphasic synovial sarcoma.

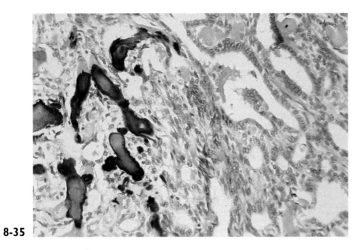

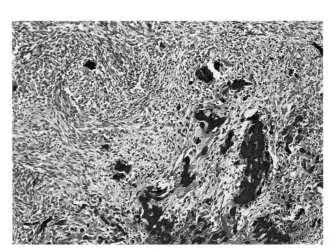

8-35

8-36

Figs. 8-35 and 8-36 Calcifications in examples of synovial sarcoma.

Synovial Sarcoma

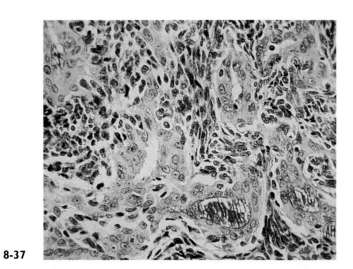

8-37

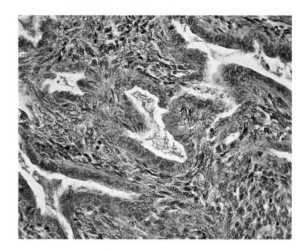

8-38

Figs. 8-37 through 8-39 PAS (Fig. 8-37) and mucicarmine stains (Figs. 8-38 and 8-39) in biphasic synovial sarcoma. Mucin is primarily intraluminal.

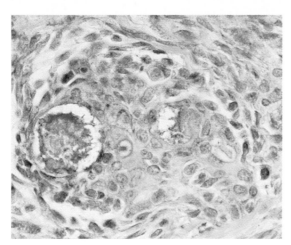

8-39

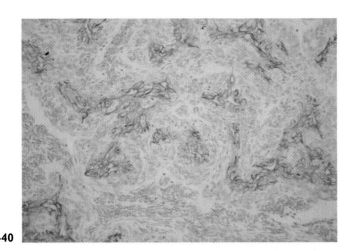

8-40

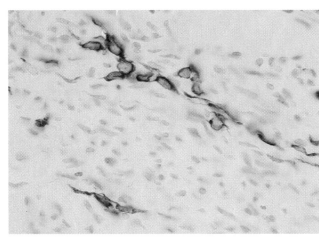

8-41

Figs. 8-40 through 8-42 Cytokeratin immunostaining in synovial sarcoma. Focal staining is typical in the spindle cell component of the fibrous type (Fig. 8-42).

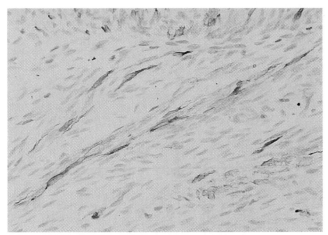

8-42

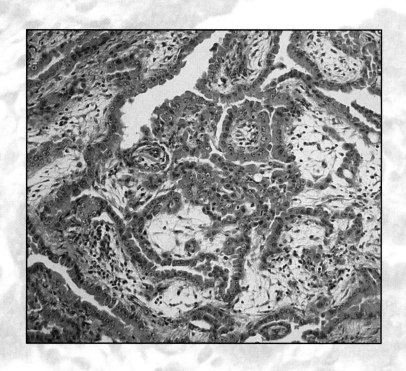

Chapter 9

Mesothelial Tumors

BENIGN

Localized Fibrous Mesothelioma (Localized Fibrous Tumor)

Localized fibrous tumor of serosal surfaces most likely arises from multipotential cells of the submesothelial fibrous connective tissue. It involves the pleura more commonly than the peritoneum, occurs in the fourth through seventh decades of life, affects women slightly more often than men, and is not clearly associated with asbestos exposure. Approximately one third of cases are reported to be associated with pulmonary osteoarthropathy, and some have been associated with hypoglycemia; otherwise they are minimally symptomatic lesions that are usually an incidental finding. Radiographically, they are well circumscribed and either pedunculated or sessile, and may be either an exophytic or endophytic growth. Histologic features cannot always be used to discriminate reliably between benign and malignant lesions; traditionally cellularity, cellular atypia, mitotic rate, size, and necrosis have been used. The prognosis of localized fibrous tumor is more closely related to the completeness of excision than to histologic features; pedunculated lesions usually have a good prognosis because they are readily excised.

MICROSCOPIC FEATURES

- Well demarcated
- Mesothelial-lined surfaces
- Cysts of varying sizes, lined by mesothelium
- Fascicular to haphazard arrangement of cells
- Uniform fibroblast-like cells
- Hypercellularity (frequently in malignant lesions)
- Nuclear hyperchromasia and atypia (malignant lesions)
- Mitoses (malignant lesions)
- Necrosis (malignant lesions)
- Collagenization
- Myxoid change
- Hemangiopericytoma-like vasculature
- Hemorrhage (variable)
- Focal calcification (variable)

DIFFERENTIAL DIAGNOSIS

- Sclerosing fibrous histiocytoma
- Hemangiopericytoma
- Fibrosarcoma
- Malignant fibrous histiocytoma
- Sarcomatoid mesothelioma
- Malignant peripheral nerve sheath tumor

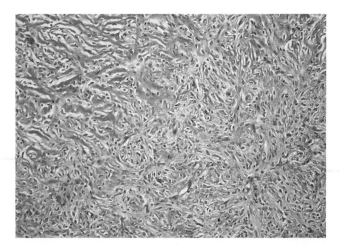

Fig. 9-1 Relatively uniform fibroblasts in a variably fibrous matrix with thin-walled vessels are seen in this localized fibrous tumor.

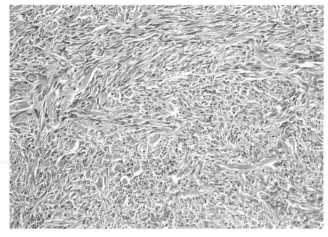

Fig. 9-2 Coarse collagen strands and mildly pleomorphic fibroblasts are seen in this example of localized fibrous tumor.

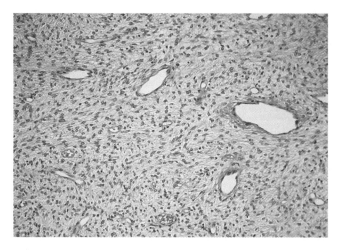

Fig. 9-3 Focally myxoid and hypocellular region with dilated vascular channels in a localized fibrous tumor.

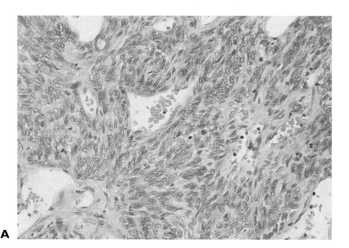

9-4A

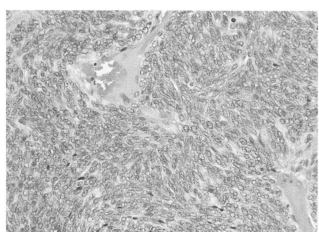

9-4B

Fig. 9-4 A and **B** An extremely cellular example of localized fibrous tumor with mitoses and atypical nuclei; probably malignant.

Multicystic Peritoneal Mesothelioma

Whether multicystic peritoneal mesothelioma is a reactive or neoplastic process is controversial, as reflected in the multiplicity of names that refer to it, including inflammatory cysts of the peritoneum; postoperative peritoneal cysts; and peritoneal, multilocular, or multicystic peritoneal inclusions cysts. It occurs primarily in young adult women, although 10% to 20% occur in men. Most frequently it presents as multiple, translucent, thin-walled cysts of varying sizes studding the visceral and parietal peritoneal surfaces. However, it may also present as a localized, multifocal mass, or a solitary mass that usually causes chronic abdominal, pelvic pain, or the sensation of a mass. Not infrequently it is associated with a history of prior abdominal or pelvic surgery, pelvic inflammatory disease, endometriosis, and/or adhesions as well as ascites. Although the lesion is histologically benign, it is frequently difficult to surgically eradicate because of the multiplicity of lesions. Approximately half of the lesions recur.

MICROSCOPIC FEATURES

- Cysts of varying sizes lined by mesothelium
- Flattened to cuboidal mesothelial cells
- "Hobnailed," eosinophilic, reactive mesothelial cells (variable)
- Papillary proliferation of mesothelial cells (variable)
- Squamous metaplasia of mesothelium (variable)
- Foci resembling adenomatoid tumor

- Bland cytologic features
- Reactive nuclear atypia (of mild to moderate degree)
- Edematous, supporting fibrous septa
- Acute and chronic inflammatory cells (in fibrous septa)
- Necrosis and fibrin (fibrous septa)
- Granulation tissue (fibrous septa)

DIFFERENTIAL DIAGNOSIS

- Cystic lymphangioma
- Microcystic adenoma of the pancreas
- Adenomatoid tumor

- Endometriosis
- Well-differentiated papillary mesothelioma
- Mesothelioma with adenomatoid foci

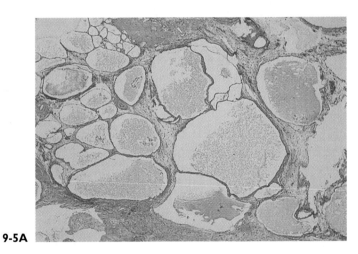
9-5A

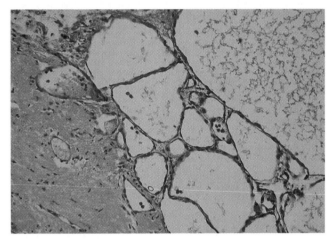
9-5B

Fig. 9-5 A and **B** Flattened mesothelial cells line cysts filled with proteinaceous fluid in this case of multicystic mesothelioma.

Adenomatoid Tumor

This distinctive, benign mesothelial proliferation is usually an incidental finding. It occurs most commonly as a solitary mass in the genital tract of men and women between 30 and 60 years of age. The lower pole of the epididymis, spermatic cord, uterus, and adnexal structures are favored sites.

MICROSCOPIC FEATURES

- Well circumscribed
- Cordlike to tubular arrangements of mesothelial cells
- Solid nests of mesothelial cells
- Flattened to cuboidal mesothelial cells
- Prominent cytoplasmic vacuoles

- Abundant eosinophilic cytoplasm
- Entrapped smooth muscle
- Fibrous stroma (variable)
- Lymphoid aggregates

DIFFERENTIAL DIAGNOSIS

- Papillary mesothelial hyperplasia
- Multicystic mesothelioma

- Well-differentiated papillary mesothelioma
- Diffuse malignant epithelial mesothelioma

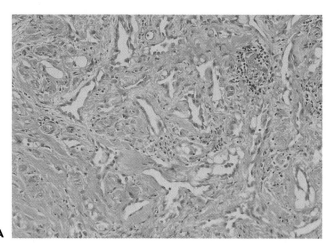
9-6A

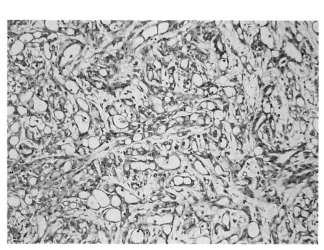
9-6B

Fig. 9-6 A and **B** Glandlike arrangements of mesothelial cells, prominent cytoplasmic vacuoles, and an abundant fibrous stroma are all seen in this case of adenomatoid tumor.

BORDERLINE

Well-Differentiated Papillary Mesothelioma

This relatively rare type of mesothelioma occurs almost exclusively in the peritoneal cavity of young women in their twenties and thirties as an incidental finding. It is characterized by the presence of multiple nodules studding the peritoneal surfaces (although solitary examples do exist), as well as a prolonged disease course with multiple local recurrences. Although the prognosis is generally favorable, occasional fatalities result from obliteration of the peritoneal cavity by tumor. This lesion is extremely well differentiated and is difficult to distinguish from papillary mesothelial hyperplasia. There is no clear association with asbestos exposure. Although some regard this tumor as a well-differentiated malignant mesothelioma, its prognosis is significantly better and, therefore, it should be regarded as a borderline or low-grade malignant lesion. The treatment is primarily surgical; the role of radiation and chemotherapy is questionable with the exception of those cases demonstrating clinical progression.

MICROSCOPIC FEATURES

- Tubulopapillary structures
- Cysts of varying sizes lined by mesothelial cells
- Solid mesothelial growth pattern
- Flattened to cuboidal mesothelial cells
- Uniform, cytologically bland mesothelial cells
- Mitoses absent (or rare)
- Psammoma bodies (variable)
- Fibrosis

DIFFERENTIAL DIAGNOSIS

- Benign papillary mesothelial hyperplasia
- Papillary serous carcinoma and borderline serous tumors of the peritoneum
- Papillary serous adenocarcinoma of the ovary
- Diffuse papillary/epithelial mesothelioma

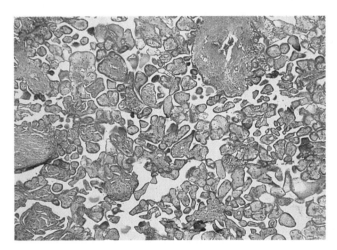

Fig. 9-7 An example of well-differentiated papillary mesothelioma that involved the peritoneal and ovarian surfaces. Note the flattened to cuboidal mesothelial cells and early cyst formation in the stroma of some of the broad papillary structures.

MALIGNANT

Malignant Localized Fibrous Mesothelioma

The histologic criteria frequently used to discriminate between benign and malignant localized fibrous tumors of the pleura and peritoneum include (1) a marked degree of hypercellularity, (2) cytologic atypia, (3) mitoses, (4) necrosis, and (5) large size. No single histologic feature is a reliable determinant of malignancy; prognosis is most closely related to completeness of excision (see Benign Localized Fibrous Mesothelioma—Discussion, Microscopic Features, Differential Diagnosis, and Captions).

Diffuse Malignant Mesothelioma

Pleural mesotheliomas outnumber peritoneal mesotheliomas by a ratio of 4:1. The overwhelming majority are diffuse as opposed to localized. Most patients with diffuse malignant mesothelioma are in the fifth through eighth decades of life, and there is a marked male predominance. Those patients with pleural involvement present with dyspnea, chest pain, cough, or fever; those with peritoneal lesions tend to have obstructive symptoms. Serous or hemorrhagic effusions or ascites are frequently seen. Mesothelioma typically presents as multiple serosal nodules that eventually coalesce to become a castlike growth that encases the viscera, causing restrictive and obstructive symptoms. This process manifests itself more prominently in the lower lobes of the lungs and diaphragm or as localized intra-abdominal masses, particularly in the omentum. Extension of the tumor into the adjacent chest or abdominal wall, diaphragm, intestines, or retro-peritoneum is not uncommon. Asbestos exposure has been reported increasingly in association with mesothelioma; this occurs primarily in patients who have worked in an asbestos-associated indus-try or lived in either an industrial or residential area contaminated with asbestos. The physical charac-teristics and type of the asbestos fibers and the

"dose" play a role in the eventual development of mesothelioma, which may have a latency period of more than 20 years from the time of exposure. The prognosis of mesothelioma is dismal, with most patients expiring within 1 to 2 years despite surgi-cal attempts at removal, including decortication. Response to radiation therapy and chemotherapy has been minimal. Metastases are most frequently to regional lymph nodes, followed by the liver, lung, adrenal glands, and bone marrow.

Diffuse mesotheliomas are divided histologically into three main types: (1) **epithelial,** (2) **fibrous (sarcomatoid),** and (3) **mixed (biphasic)** types. The predominantly epithelial type reportedly accounts for 70% to 75% of diffuse mesotheliomas, but in reality, most lesions constitute a spectrum with overlapping features, although relatively pure forms may be seen. Predominantly fibrous types have an especially poor prognosis.

Epithelial Mesothelioma

MICROSCOPIC FEATURES

- Tubulopapillary pattern
- Solid nests or sheets of cells
- Irregular to microcystic spaces
- Flattened to cuboidal mesothelial cells
- Abundant eosinophilic cytoplasm, sometimes finely vacuolated or glassy
- Prominent cytoplasmic vacuoles (reminiscent of adenomatoid tumor)
- Intracellular glycogen
- Extracellular and intracellular mucin, hyaluronidase-sensitive
- Uniform, round nuclei
- Prominent nucleoli
- Mitoses
- Freely floating, single cells in mucinous pools or cysts
- Psammomatous calcifications (variable)

Fibrous (Sarcomatoid) Mesothelioma

MICROSCOPIC FEATURES

- Whorled to hemangiopericytic pattern (variable)
- Fascicles
- Spindled cells resembling fibroblasts
- Nuclear hyperchromasia and atypia
- Hyalinization (variable)
- Myxoid stroma (rare)
- Osseous and/or chondroid metaplasia (rare)
- Epithelial foci (rare)

Biphasic Mesothelioma

MICROSCOPIC FEATURES

- Admixture of epithelial and sarcomatoid elements (see Epithelial and Fibrous/Sarcomatoid

Mesothelioma, p. 207)

All Malignant Mesotheliomas

DIFFERENTIAL DIAGNOSIS

- Reactive mesothelial hyperplasia
- Multicystic peritoneal mesothelioma
- Well-differentiated papillary mesothelioma
- Synovial sarcoma
- Carcinosarcoma (other organ systems)
- Fibrosarcoma

- Malignant fibrous histiocytoma
- Malignant peripheral nerve sheath tumor
- Metastatic papillary adenocarcinoma, especially of ovarian origin
- Papillary serous carcinoma and borderline serous tumors of the peritoneum

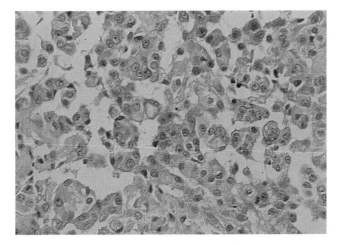

Fig. 9-8 A predominantly epithelial mesothelioma in a female presenting as a periumbilical mass. The tubulopapillary pattern predominates. The cells are cuboidal with uniform, prominent nucleoli.

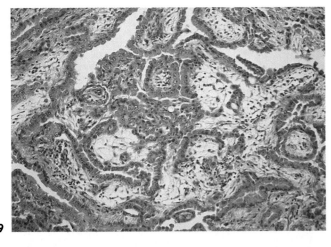

9-9

Figs. 9-9 and 9-10 A and **B** Examples of biphasic mesotheliomas. The epithelioid elements are prominent.

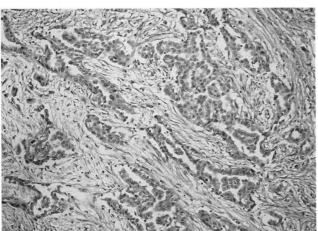

-10A

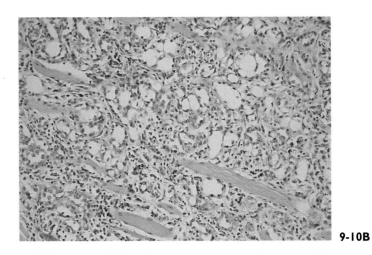

9-10B

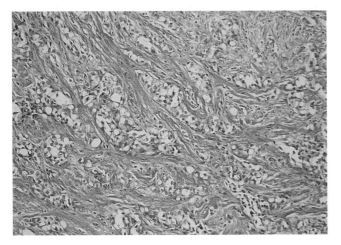

Fig. 9-11 Mesothelioma with areas resembling an adenomatoid tumor.

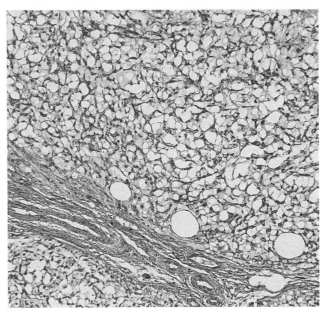

Fig. 9-12 Mesothelioma with sheets of clear cells resulting in an appearance similar to an adenomatoid tumor.

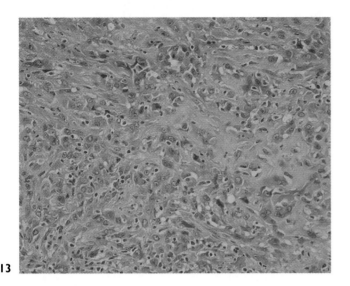

9-13

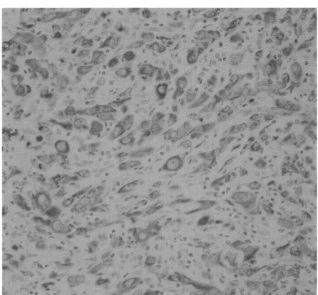

9-14

Figs. 9-13 and 9-14 A mesothelioma with spindled and epithelioid areas that stained strongly for keratin (Fig. 9-14). Notice the focally prominent hyalinized matrix.

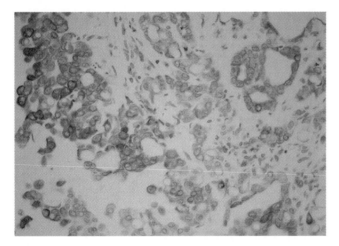

Fig. 9-15 Mesothelioma showing typical staining pattern of epithelioid cells for cytokeratin.

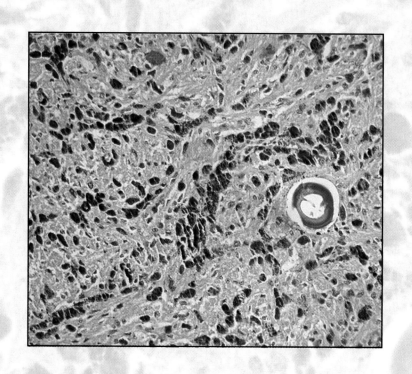

Chapter 10

Neuroectodermal Tumors

BENIGN

Traumatic Neuroma

This lesion is a painful, reparative process emanating from the proximal end of a nerve trunk that has been severed and not properly aligned with its distal end. It occurs after surgery or trauma, frequently after amputation.

MICROSCOPIC FEATURES

- Circumscribed
- Disorderly arrangement of nerve fascicles
- Admixture of fibroblasts, Schwann cells, and axons
- Fibrous matrix
- Myxoid change (variable)

DIFFERENTIAL DIAGNOSIS

- Scar
- Morton's neuroma
- Neurofibroma

Morton's Neuroma

This reactive, sclerosing process is closely associated with peripheral nerves located in the second, third, and fourth metatarsal heads, and less commonly the hands. Women are affected more often than men. Repeated minor trauma is a likely etiologic factor.

MICROSCOPIC FEATURES

- Ill defined margins
- Extension of fibrosis to adjacent soft tissue and vessel walls (variable)
- Irregular distribution of elastic fibrils
- Perineural fibrosis

DIFFERENTIAL DIAGNOSIS

- Scar
- Traumatic neuroma
- Neurofibroma

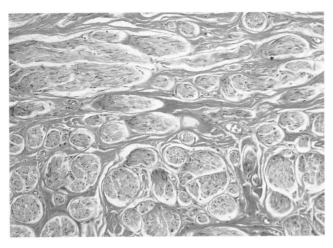

Fig. 10-1 Example of a neuroma in which perineural fibrosis is prominent.

Nerve Sheath Ganglion

Nerve sheath ganglion most likely represents a degenerative process that consists of a ganglion cyst–like structure arising within the confines of a nerve trunk. Most frequently it is associated with the popliteal nerve.

MICROSCOPIC FEATURES

- Cyst formation, frequently at periphery of nerve
- Mucinous material within the cyst
- No cyst lining

DIFFERENTIAL DIAGNOSIS

- Ganglion cyst
- Myxoma
- Juxta-articular myxoma
- Neurothekeoma (nerve sheath myxoma)

Neuromuscular Hamartoma (Benign Triton Tumor)

This extremely rare lesion occurs at any age and is associated with peripheral nerves. It is believed to be a hamartoma and may possibly arise from a maldeveloped limb bud.

MICROSCOPIC FEATURES

- Epineural circumscription and perineural septal compartmentalization
- Well-differentiated skeletal muscle arranged in bundles and replacing peripheral nerves
- Multilobular architecture
- Axons, myelinated and nonmyelinated, arranged in fascicles
- Fibromatosis-like proliferation (variable)

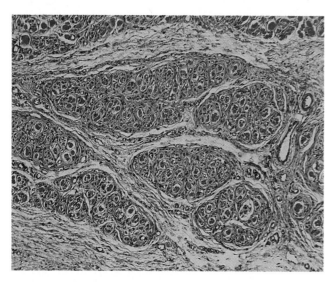

Fig. 10-2 Low magnification of a cross section of a benign Triton tumor showing compartmentalization by epineural and perineural fibrous connective tissue.

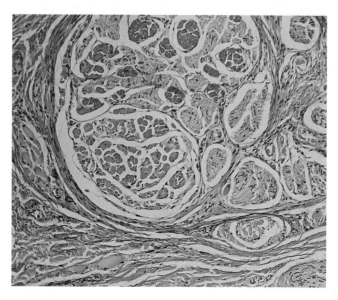

Fig. 10-3 Slender skeletal muscle fibers are intimately associated with peripheral nerves. Both components are surrounded by the epineurium and its ramifications.

Schwannoma (Neurilemoma)

Schwannomas are benign peripheral nerve sheath tumors composed almost exclusively of Schwann cells. They occur as either superficial or deep solitary masses in men or women in the third through sixth decades of life, although multiple central nervous system lesions may be seen in the central form of neurofibromatosis. Schwannomas are slowly growing masses that may be present for years; they have a proclivity to involve the head and neck, extremities, mediastinum, and retroperitoneum.

Pain is uncommon, and symptoms are attributable to pressure on adjacent structures. They rarely recur even when incompletely excised. The **cellular schwannoma,** which consists almost exclusively of Antoni A areas, deserves special mention because it may be easily confused with a malignant peripheral nerve sheath tumor, particularly in biopsies. Deep-seated schwannomas are more likely to display secondary degenerative changes. **Plexiform schwannomas** are not associated with neurofibromatosis.

MICROSCOPIC FEATURES

- Encapsulated
- Eccentric location in a nerve trunk
- Plexiform/multinodular pattern (rare)
- Short fascicles or swirls
- Nuclear palisading (Verocay bodies)
- Compact cellular zones (Antoni A areas)
- Rarefied, hypocellular zones (Antoni B areas)
- Spindled to oval to angulated nuclei
- Mild nuclear pleomorphism
- Nuclear hyperchromasia
- Intranuclear cytoplasmic invaginations or vacuoles

- Mitoses (variable)
- Ill-defined cytoplasmic margins (syncytial arrangement of cells)
- Eosinophilic, homogeneous to finely fibrillary cytoplasm, similar to neuropil
- Myxoid change (primarily Antoni B areas)
- Degenerative or reactive changes, including: Hemorrhage, fibrin, organizing thrombi, hemosiderin deposition, xanthoma cells, lymphoid aggregates, cyst formation, necrosis, calcification, extreme hyalinization, vessels with hyalinized walls

DIFFERENTIAL DIAGNOSIS

- Organizing thrombus
- Nonspecific fibrosis
- Neurofibroma
- Leiomyoma

- Malignant peripheral nerve sheath tumor
- Melanoma
- Leiomyosarcoma

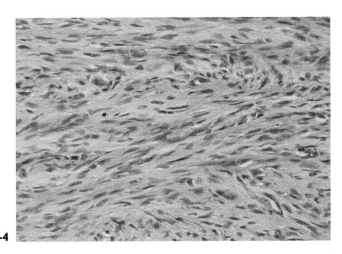
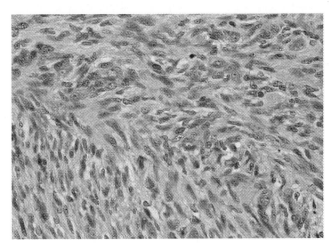

10-4   10-5

Figs. 10-4 and 10-5 Nuclear hyperchromasia and mild nuclear pleomorphism are characteristic features of benign schwannomas. Areas of increased cellularity may also be seen (Fig. 10-5).

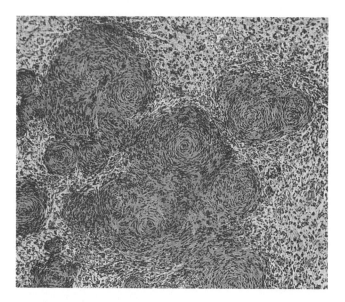

Fig. 10-6 Whorled Antoni A areas may be seen in schwannomas.

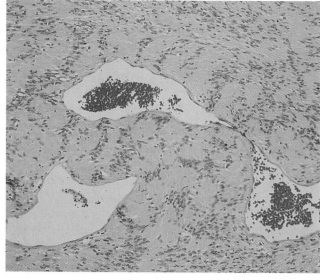

Fig. 10-7 Prominent palisading is seen in this schwannoma.

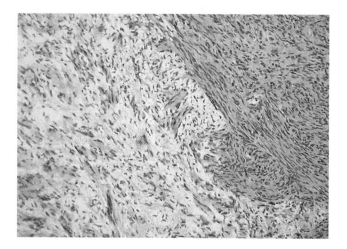

Fig. 10-8 Hypocellular Antoni B areas apposed to Antoni A areas.

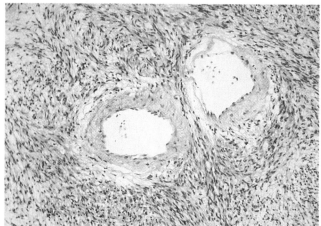

Fig. 10-9 Thick-walled hyalinized blood vessels are another characteristic feature of schwannoma.

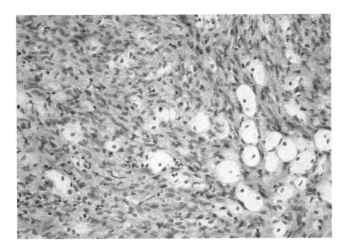

Fig. 10-10 Clusters of xanthoma cells may be prominent in schwannoma.

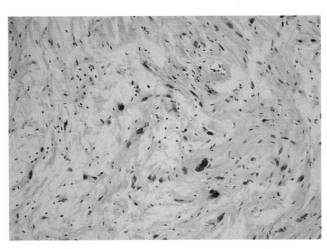

Fig. 10-11 Nuclear pleomorphism and hyperchromasia in a schwannoma.

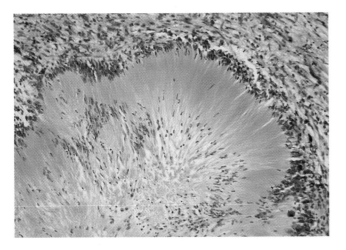

Fig. 10-12 Example of palisading around a collagen core seen in schwannoma.

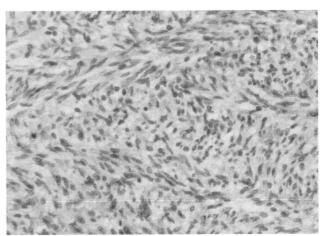

Fig. 10-13 S100 protein immunostaining in schwannomas is typically intense and diffuse.

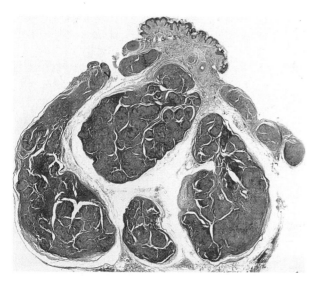

Fig. 10-14 A schwannoma with a plexiform or multinodular architecture (plexiform schwannoma) occurring in the subcutis. These lesions should not be confused with plexiform neurofibroma or plexiform malignant peripheral nerve sheath tumor, nor should they be construed as evidence of neurofibromatosis.

Neurothekeoma (Nerve Sheath Myxoma)

Neurothekeoma is a superficial neural neoplasm that tends to occur in the head and neck, upper trunk, and fingers of young adults. Most involve the dermis or subcutis; they are occasionally associated with a nerve trunk or a neurofibroma. Local recurrences are rare. Ultrastructural and immunohistochemical studies have displayed features of Schwann and perineurial nerve sheath cells.

MICROSCOPIC FEATURES

- Multilobular architecture
- Packeted arrangement of cells with fibrous septa
- Whorled arrangement of cells within packets
- Relatively uniform, round to spindled cells
- Epithelioid to histiocytoid cells (variable)
- Mitoses (variable)
- Hypercellular areas (variable)
- Prominent myxoid matrix

DIFFERENTIAL DIAGNOSIS

- Mucinosis
- Myxoma
- Myxoid neurofibroma
- Myxoid malignant fibrous histiocytoma

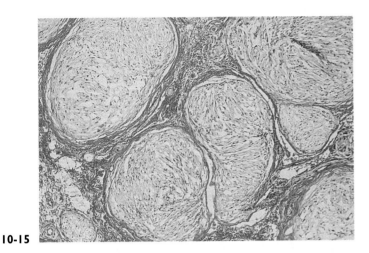

10-15

Figs. 10-15 and 10-16 A and B (A) Neurothekeomas demonstrating packeted arrangements of cells, a prominent myxoid matrix, fibrous septa, and variably rounded to spindled, mildly pleomorphic cells. **(B)** Example of cellular neurothekeoma that bears a resemblance to various sarcomas.

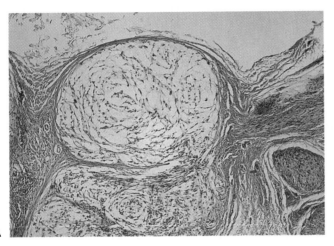

0-16A

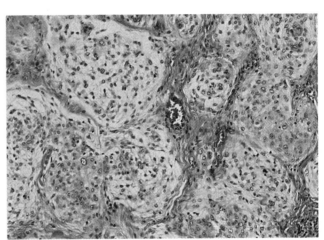

10-16B

Neurofibroma

Neurofibromas are peripheral nerve sheath tumors that, in contrast to schwannomas, consist of an admixture of cells, primarily Schwann cells, as well as variable numbers of fibroblasts, axonal processes of neurons, and probably perineurial nerve sheath cells. There are a variety of types of neurofibromas. By far the most common type is the **localized neurofibroma,** which is frequently myxoid; the majority of these occur outside the setting of von Recklinghausen's disease (NF-1), but multiple localized neurofibromas may be seen in NF-1 as well. Localized neurofibromas outside the setting of NF-1 tend to affect the sexes equally and have a peak incidence in the third decade of life. Most are superficial, painless lesions that tend to occur in the subcutis and dermis; origin from a nerve trunk may be seen. Localized neurofibromas arising within

NF-1 are usually multiple, superficially or deeply located, frequently larger, and more likely to undergo malignant degeneration.

Pacinian, epithelioid, and pigmented neurofibromas are best regarded as unusual variants of localized neurofibroma. **Pacinian neurofibromas** more or less recapitulate the histologic appearance of pressure receptors with a targetoid or onionskin-like growth pattern. They tend to involve the distal extremities and buttocks in adolescents and adults; there is no known association with von Recklinghausen's disease.

Epithelioid neurofibroma is distinguished by the presence of epithelioid cells that are arranged in nests and cords. Although it is probably clinically not significant, it is histologically difficult to recognize as being neural in origin unless it is associated with a nerve trunk or neurofibroma.

Pigmented neurofibromas are also rare. Other than the presence of melanin in the cytoplasm of lesional cells, they are otherwise morphologically similar to the solitary neurofibroma.

Diffuse neurofibroma is a superficially and ill-defined variant of neurofibroma that occurs as a solitary mass in children and adolescents. Approximately 10% are associated with von Recklinghausen's disease.

Plexiform neurofibroma refers to diffuse enlargement and distortion of a major nerve trunk by a disorganized growth of nerves within and occasionally also outside the nerve trunk. Giant, severely disfiguring examples of plexiform neurofibroma involving a large area of the body and sometimes associated pigmentation of the overlying skin have been referred to as elephantiasis neuromatosa. Plexiform neurofibromas are most frequently seen in association with NF-1; while their presence suggests von Recklinghausen's disease, as an isolated finding they are not pathognomonic for NF-1.

Although all neurofibromas may undergo malignant degeneration, those that arise in patients with von Recklinghausen's disease carry a significantly higher risk of malignant transformation over a long time. Malignant peripheral nerve sheath tumors arising in patients with von Recklinghausen's disease also have an especially poor prognosis.

Localized Neurofibroma and Its Variants

MICROSCOPIC FEATURES

- Encapsulation (variable)
- Fusiform expansion of a nerve trunk (variable)
- Fascicles, whorls, or a storiform pattern
- Nests and cords (epithelioid neurofibroma)
- Tactoid structures resembling Wagner-Meissner complexes
- Concentric structures resembling pacinian bodies (pacinian neurofibroma)
- Elongated cells with wiry, eosinophilic processes
- Epithelioid cells (epithelioid variant of neurofibroma)
- Melanin pigment (pigmented neurofibroma)
- Serpentine, wavy, comma-shaped, or buckled nuclei
- Hyperchromatic nuclei
- Mast cells
- Lymphocytes (variable)
- Xanthoma cells (rare)
- Myxoid matrix (myxoid neurofibroma)
- Hyalinization

Diffuse Neurofibroma

MICROSCOPIC FEATURES

- Ill-defined margins
- Infiltrative, nondestructive growth pattern in dermis and subcutis
- Delicate collagen fibrils
- Round to oval to serpentine nuclei
- Tactoid structures resembling Wagner-Meissner corpuscles
- Nuclear palisading (variable)
- Associated with other mesenchymal elements such as adipose tissue or blood vessels (rare)

Plexiform Neurofibroma

MICROSCOPIC FEATURES

- Disorganized proliferation of Schwann cells and fibroblasts within the perineurial confines and sometimes outside the perineurium
- Elongated Schwann cells with serpentine, wavy nuclei

- Entrapped axons
- Nuclear pleomorphism (variable)
- Mitoses (rare, suggestive of malignant degeneration)
- Collagen fibrils
- Myxoid matrix

All Neurofibromas

DIFFERENTIAL DIAGNOSIS

- Schwannoma
- Fibrous histiocytoma
- Plexiform fibrohistiocytic tumor (plexiform neurofibroma)
- Myxoma
- Blue nevus and cellular blue nevus

- Dermatofibrosarcoma protuberans
- Bednar tumor (pigmented dermatofibrosarcoma protuberans)
- Malignant peripheral nerve sheath tumor (MPNST)
- Spindle cell or desmoplastic melanoma

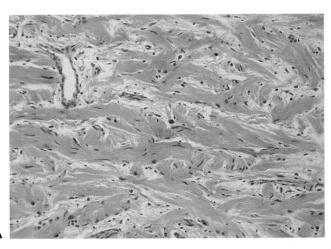

10-17A

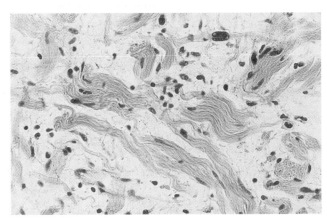

10-17B

Fig. 10-17 A and **B** Microscopic appearances of neurofibromas in which the cells have delicate, wiry to thick eosinophilic processes and a variable amount of collagen deposition. Notice the characteristic serpentine shape of the nuclei and slight nuclear pleomorphism.

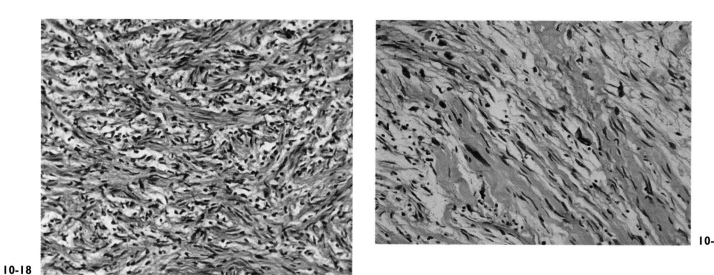

10-18

10-19

Figs. 10-18 and 10-19 Neurofibromas may have hypercellular areas and focally pleomorphic, hyperchromatic nuclei, especially when they occur in patients with von Recklinghausen's disease or in a plexiform neurofibroma. Some of these cases have been designated pleomorphic neurofibroma and neurofibroma with degenerative atypia. Such changes should not be misinterpreted as evidence of malignant degeneration, but a marked increase in cellularity should prompt a search for mitotic figures and necrosis (i.e., evidence of malignant degeneration).

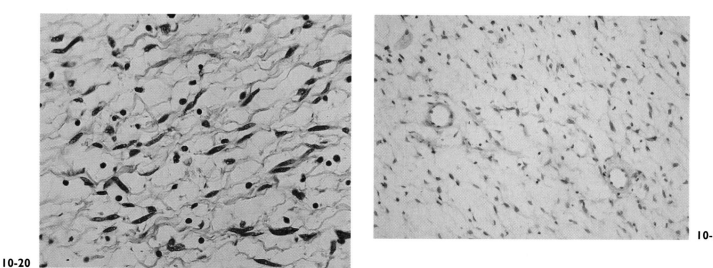

10-20

10-21

Figs. 10-20 and 10-21 Neurofibromas with a prominent myxoid matrix are commonly referred to as myxoid neurofibroma.

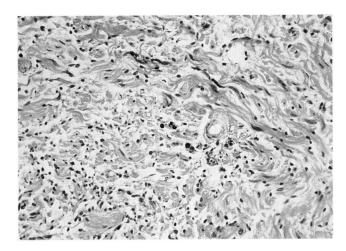

Fig. 10-22 Melanin pigment distinguishes the pigmented neurofibroma from its more conventional counterpart.

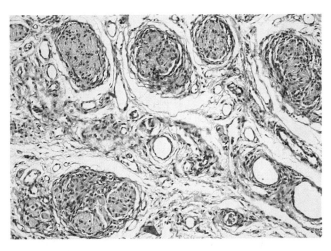

Fig. 10-23 Example of pacinian neurofibroma showing a whorled appearance and a resemblance to pressure receptors.

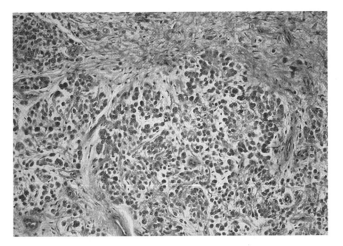

Fig. 10-24 Typical example of epithelioid neurofibroma in which the cells are plump with abundant eosinophilic cytoplasm. A cord-like arrangement of cells may be seen in some epithelioid neurofibromas.

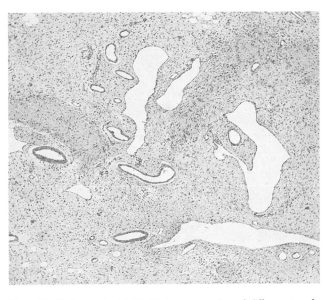

10-25

Figs. 10-25 through 10-29 Various examples of diffuse neurofibroma showing Wagner-Meissner corpuscle–like structures amid a diffuse background of infiltrating small, round to spindled neuroid cells. Involvement of skeletal muscle by diffuse neurofibroma occasionally may be seen. Immunostains for S100 protein usually stain the Wagner-Meissner body–like structures (Fig. 10-29, S100 protein).

(Figs continued on next page.)

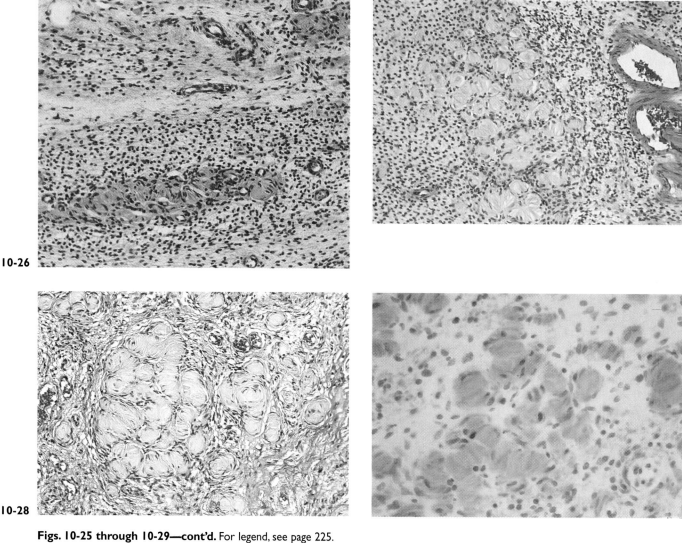

10-26

10-2

10-28

10-29

Figs. 10-25 through 10-29—cont'd. For legend, see page 225.

Granular Cell Tumor

Granular cell tumor is a fairly common lesion that tends to present as a superficial, solitary mass in adults during the fourth through sixth decades of life. The tongue is the most common site, followed by the chest wall and arms. Local recurrence is rare in benign lesions. The overwhelming majority of granular cell tumors are benign, but the histologic criteria to distinguish benign and malignant granular cell tumors are not well defined, and perfectly benign-appearing granular cell tumors have on rare occasions metastasized.

MICROSCOPIC FEATURES

- Poorly circumscribed to infiltrative growth pattern
- Nests, strands, cords, and sheets
- Intimate association with nerves (variable)
- Round to polygonal cells
- Abundant, coarse, eosinophilic cytoplasmic granules
- Uniform, central nuclei
- Minimal nuclear pleomorphism
- Mitoses (rare)
- Fibrosis or desmoplasia (variable)
- Pseudoepitheliomatous hyperplasia of overlying squamous epithelium

Neuroectodermal Tumors

DIFFERENTIAL DIAGNOSIS

- Reactive granular cell change in scars or foreign body granulomas
- Adult rhabdomyoma
- Hibernoma
- Paraganglioma
- Malignant granular cell tumor

- Secondary granular cell change in neoplasms such as: fibrous histiocytoma, leiomyoma, leiomyosarcoma, and angiosarcoma
- Alveolar soft part sarcoma
- Squamous carcinoma

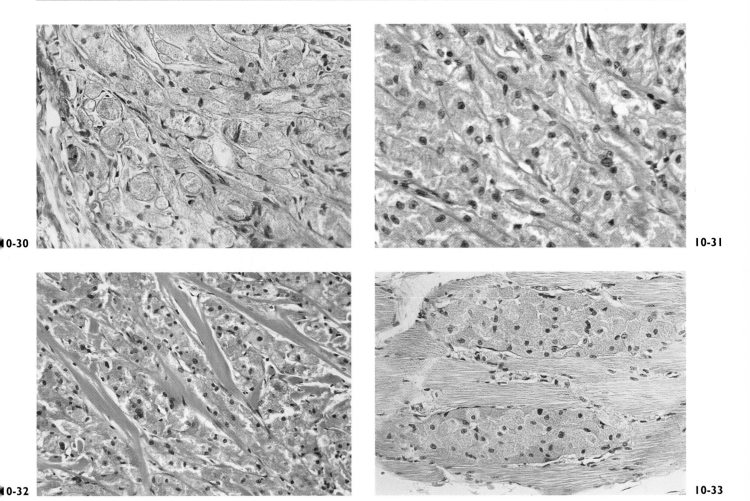

10-30

10-31

10-32

10-33

Figs. 10-30 through 10-34 Various examples of granular cell tumor with a benign histologic appearance. Some cases may infiltrate skeletal muscle or be associated with fibrosis, desmoplasia, or lymphoid aggregates.

(Figs continued on next page.)

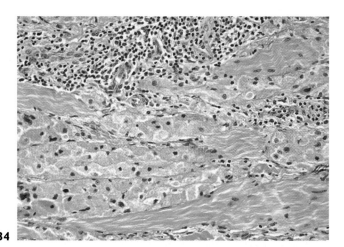

10-34

Figs. 10-30 through 10-34—cont'd. For legend, see page 227.

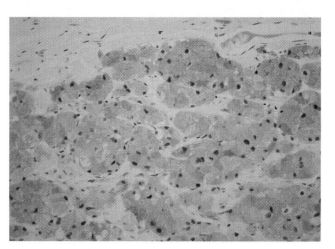

Fig. 10-35 S100 protein immunostaining in a granular cell tumor.

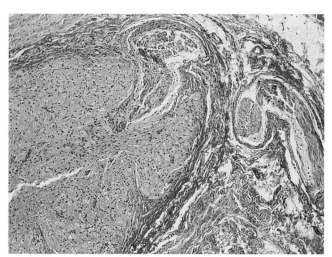

Fig. 10-36 Granular cell tumor showing intimate association with a peripheral nerve.

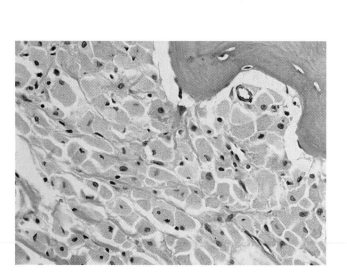

Fig. 10-37 Example of reactive granular cell proliferation that bears a close resemblance to granular cell tumor.

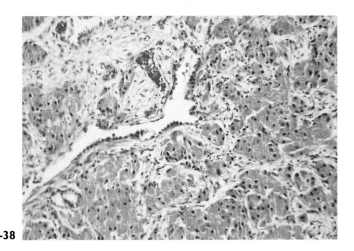

10-38

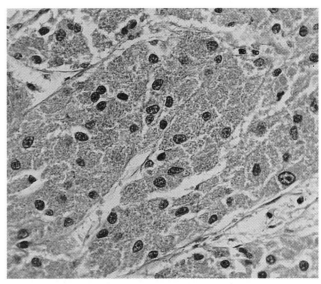

10-39

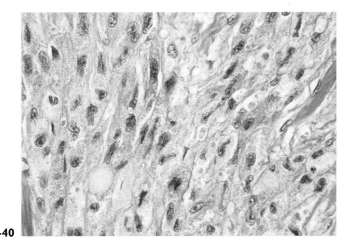

10-40

Figs. 10-38 through 10-40 Examples of malignant granular cell tumor that metastasized. Although these tumors are similar to benign granular cell tumors, the cells have a higher nuclear/cytoplasmic ratio, prominent nucleoli, and display a spindled pattern in some areas. Mitotic activity is usually more prominent than in benign granular cell tumors.

Melanotic Schwannoma

This unusual type of schwannoma occurs primarily in adults, usually along the vertebral axis, and is frequently associated with autonomic or sympathetic nerves. A unique subgroup termed *psammomatous melanotic schwannoma,* characterized by the presence of melanin, fat, and psammoma bodies, has been described. Psammomatous melanotic schwannoma is a relatively indolent, slowly growing lesion that is clinically distinctive because of its association in over half the cases with Carney's complex (consisting of myxomas, spotty pigmentation, and endocrine overactivity), which is transmitted as an autosomal dominant trait.

Patients with the complex tend to present 10 years younger with melanotic schwannomas than those without the complex. Approximately 20% of these schwannomas are multiple; they frequently involve posterior spinal nerve roots, the gastrointestinal tract, and sometimes bone. About 15% of patients have died from their tumors, usually due to metastases, which are most frequently to lungs and pleura. Other than metastases, reliable criteria to distinguish benign from malignant lesions are not well defined (see Malignant Melanotic Schwannoma). The proportion of melanotic schwannomas composed of the calcifying/psammomatous type is unknown.

MICROSCOPIC FEATURES

- Well circumscribed
- Schwannoma-like cellular proliferation
- Fusiform to round, vesicular, hyperchromatic nuclei
- Multinucleated cells
- Prominent nucleoli
- Intranuclear cytoplasmic vacuoles

- Mitoses (variable)
- Heavy pigmentation with melanin
- Psammomatous calcifications that frequently coalesce
- Adipose tissue
- Degenerative changes similar to benign schwannoma
- Lymphocytic aggregates

DIFFERENTIAL DIAGNOSIS

- Pigmented neurofibroma
- Pigmented meningioma
- Melanoma (balloon cell, acral lentiginous, and desmoplastic types)

- Schwannoma
- Malignant peripheral nerve sheath tumor
- Clear cell sarcoma

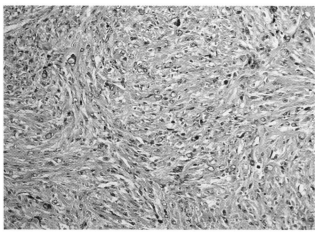

10-41

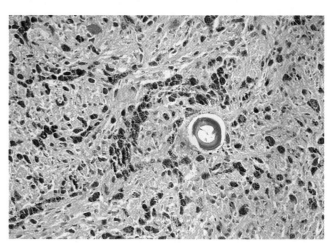

10-42

Figs. 10-41 and 10-42 A case of melanotic schwannoma demonstrating a syncytium of pleomorphic Schwann cells interspersed with abundant melanin pigment and rare calcifications. Iron deposition is seen focally.

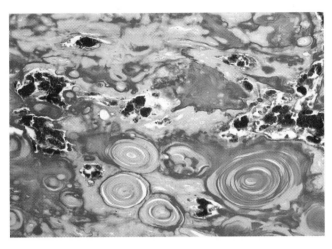

Fig. 10-43 Coalescing psammomatous calcifications characterize this unique variant of melanotic schwannoma.

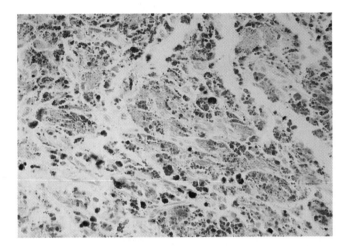

Fig. 10-44 Iron stain demonstrating iron (blue) and abundant melanin (brown) in a melanotic schwannoma.

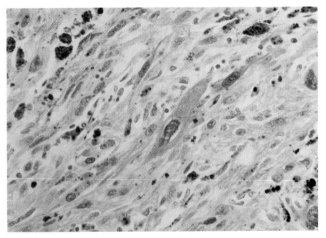

Fig. 10-45 S100 protein immunostaining is seen in melanotic schwannoma.

Ganglioneuroma

By definition, ganglioneuroma does not possess immature elements. Most cases probably arise de novo, although a few may represent ganglioneuroblastomas that have matured. Most patients are 10 years old or older, with the majority of lesions occurring in the mediastinum and retroperitoneum. They may arise occasionally in association with pheochromocytoma. Some cases are associated with the production of vasoactive intestinal peptide and resultant diarrhea. Transformation of ganglioneuroma to malignant peripheral nerve sheath tumor is rare.

MICROSCOPIC FEATURES

- Well-circumscribed with a fibrous capsule
- Intersecting fascicles of Schwann cells resembling neurofibroma
- Nests of or isolated ganglion cells
- Mature ganglion cells, occasionally multinucleated

DIFFERENTIAL DIAGNOSIS

- Neurofibroma
- Proliferative fasciitis and myositis
- Ganglioneuroblastoma
- Malignant peripheral nerve sheath tumor
- Ectomesenchymoma

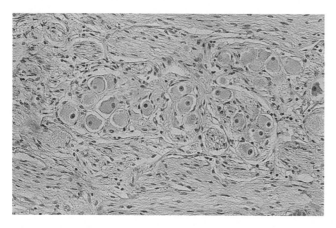

Fig. 10-46 Example of a ganglioneuroma showing clusters of ganglion cells in a background of mature neurofibroma-like tissue.

Ectopic Meningioma

Extracranial meningioma by definition is not associated with, or an extension of, an intracranial meningioma. It occurs most commonly in the skin and soft tissues of the scalp and paravertebral region, and most likely arises from nests of arachnoid cells residing in the subcutis secondary to a defect in neural tube closure or along the pathways of sensory nerves of the eye, ear, and nose. There is a bimodal age distribution; those arising in children and young adults are more likely to be cystic, and those arising primarily in adults more closely recapitulate the appearance of intracranial meningioma.

MICROSCOPIC FEATURES

- Whorls, nests, and sheets of meningothelial cells
- Cysts (variable)
- Psammomatous calcifications
- Collagen (variable)

DIFFERENTIAL DIAGNOSIS

- Intracranial meningioma

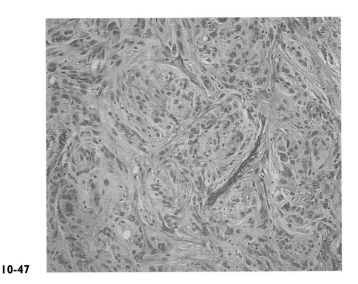

10-47

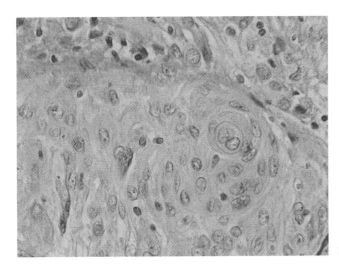

10-48

Figs. 10-47 and 10-48 Examples of extracranial meningioma with nests of meningothelial cells associated with variable amounts of collagen.

Pigmented Neuroectodermal Tumor Of Infancy (Retinal Anlage Tumor, Progonoma)

This unusual, primitive, pigmented, neuroepithelial neoplasm is believed to be of neural crest origin. It typically occurs in infants less than 1 year of age and classically presents in the upper or lower jaw as a destructive, radiolucent lesion. Less commonly, the epididymis, mediastinum, brain, and anterior fontanelle are involved. Approximately 15% of cases recur locally, and a small percentage metastasize. Criteria (other than metastases) to distinguish benign from malignant lesions are not well defined. The neuroepithelial and melanocytic nature of these lesions has been well documented both ultrastructurally and immunohistochemically.

MICROSCOPIC FEATURES

- Multicystic lesion
- Cystic spaces lined by primitive, cuboidal, pigmented cells
- Primitive neuroblastoma-like cells within cystic spaces
- Neuropil-like stroma associated with primitive cells
- Ganglioneuroma-like foci
- Fibrous stroma between cysts

DIFFERENTIAL DIAGNOSIS

- Neuroblastoma
- Ganglioneuroblastoma
- Primitive neuroectodermal tumor
- Melanoma
- Rhabdomyosarcoma

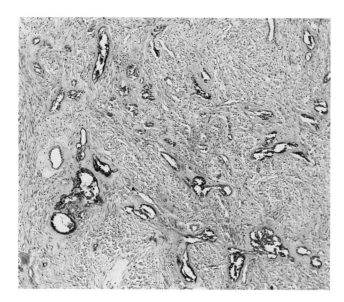

Fig. 10-49 A rather fibrous, pigmented neuroectodermal tumor of infancy, with primitive neuroepithelial and pigmented cells lining cystic areas.

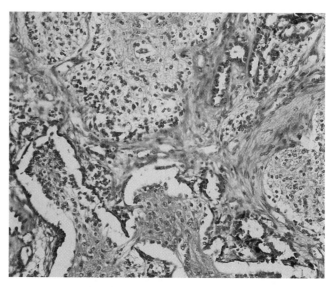

Fig. 10-50 A pigmented neuroectodermal tumor of infancy demonstrating nodular foci of primitive neuroepithelial cells in a neuropil-like stroma and surrounded by cuboidal pigmented cells containing melanin. Note the close resemblance of the lesion to a neuroblastoma. The intervening stroma is fibrous.

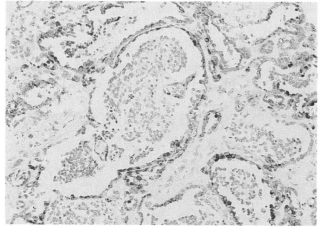

10-51

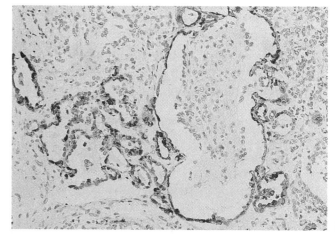

10-52

Figs. 10-51 and 10-52 Cytokeratin (Fig. 10-51) and HMB45 (Fig. 10-52) stain the pigmented lining cells of a pigmented neuroectodermal tumor of infancy.

MALIGNANT

Malignant Peripheral Nerve Sheath Tumor (Malignant Schwannoma)

The criteria for the diagnosis of MPNST vary, and therefore comparison of various studies is not always possible. Traditional criteria have stated that the lesion must arise in a nerve trunk, a neurofibroma, or a patient with von Recklinghausen's disease. However, some sarcomas do not meet these criteria but are morphologically indistinguishable from those that do. Therefore the criteria to diagnose MPNST have become less stringent over time and are now primarily morphologic, acknowledging that poorly differentiated MPNST unassociated with the aforementioned criteria will not be recognized.

Using less stringent criteria, approximately 50% of cases of MPNST arise in patients with von Recklinghausen's disease, usually after a latency period of 10 to 20 years. Moreover, MPNST in patients with neurofibromatosis may be multicentric (particularly in plexiform neurofibromas) or multiple. MPNST is primarily a tumor of adults, although patients with neurofibromatosis may present with malignancy at a younger age. In sporadic cases of MPNST the sex ratio is approximately equal, whereas in von Recklinghausen's disease there is a 4:1 male predominance. MPNST has a proclivity to occur in the proximal limbs and trunk. Symptoms of nerve compression are characteristic, and pain or rapid enlargement of a neurofibroma in a patient with neurofibromatosis may herald malignant transformation. The survival rate is lower in patients with neurofibromatosis, which appears to be an independent adverse prognostic factor. Tumor size (stage) and location also undoubtedly affect prognosis. Metastases are usually to lungs, liver, subcutis, and bone. Lymph node metastases are rare.

MPNST may display divergent differentiation (heterologous components). The more commonly recognized types include those with **rhabdomyoblastic** differentiation (**malignant Triton tumor**) and benign or malignant **glands** (MPNST with **glandular differentiation**). MPNST also commonly displays varying degrees of chondroid and/or osseous differentiation; these components may exhibit bland or malignant histologic features. Reports regarding the behavior of MPNST with divergent differentiation, particularly with regard to malignant Triton tumors, are contradictory. The preponderance of evidence to date suggests that they behave similar to other MPNSTs.

Malignant epithelioid schwannoma also merits separate mention because it may be difficult to distinguish from malignant epithelial, melanocytic, and other mesenchymal neoplasms unless it is associated with areas of typical MPNST or associated with a nerve trunk or neurofibroma. Its prognosis is similar to other MPNST.

Malignant Peripheral Nerve Sheath Tumor

MICROSCOPIC FEATURES

- Well-circumscribed to multinodular
- Fascicles resembling fibrosarcoma
- Whorls
- Sharply demarcated hypercellular and hypocellular zones (marbled appearance)
- Elongated cells with wavy, serpentine, angulated, nuclei
- Round to oval nuclei
- Mild nuclear pleomorphism
- Mitoses
- Primitive neuroepithelial-like foci (rare)
- Fibrillary cytoplasm (variable)

- Tactoid structures (rare)
- Nuclear palisading
- Vascular luminal herniation
- Rosettes (rare)
- Hemangiopericytic vascular pattern
- Perivascular targetoid growth pattern
- Fibrosis (variable)
- Myxoid matrix
- Geographic zones of tumor necrosis with perivascular tumor cell preservation
- Heterologous elements such as: bone, cartilage, skeletal muscle, epithelium (glandular or squamous)

Malignant Epithelioid Schwannoma

MICROSCOPIC FEATURES

- Multinodular or vaguely nodular architecture
- Cords and nests of cells
- Polygonal to epithelioid cells
- Relatively round nuclei with prominent nucleoli

- Variable amount of clear to eosinophilic cytoplasm
- Myxoid matrix
- Areas of conventional MPNST

All Malignant Peripheral Nerve Sheath Tumors (MPNST)

DIFFERENTIAL DIAGNOSIS

- Cellular schwannoma
- Pleomorphic, cellular neurofibroma
- Epithelioid neurofibroma
- Leiomyosarcoma
- Fibrosarcoma
- Synovial sarcoma

- Hemangiopericytoma
- Clear cell sarcoma (melanoma of soft parts)
- Melanoma, especially neurotropic melanoma
- Peripheral neuroepithelioma
- Carcinoma

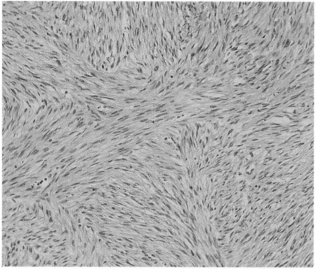

10-53

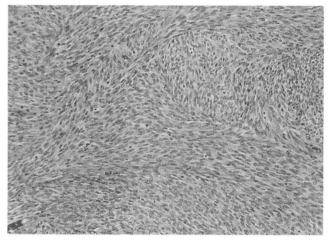

10-54

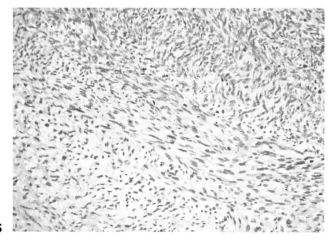

10-55

Figs. 10-53 through 10-55 A fascicular to focally storiform pattern is frequently seen in malignant peripheral nerve sheath tumors, creating a close resemblance to fibrosarcoma. The matrix is variably myxoid to fibrous. In general, the cells of malignant peripheral nerve sheath tumor are slender, fusiform, and serpentine.

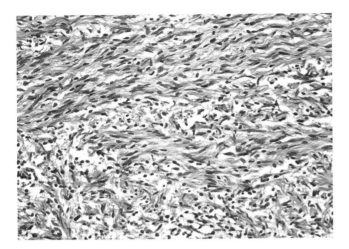

Fig. 10-56 A malignant peripheral nerve sheath tumor with a neurofibroma-like appearance showing characteristic serpentine nuclei.

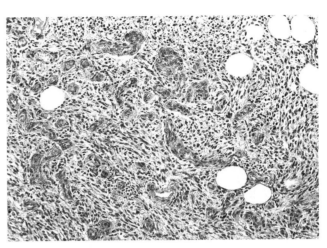

Fig. 10-57 A malignant peripheral nerve sheath tumor with proliferation of plump endothelial lining cells.

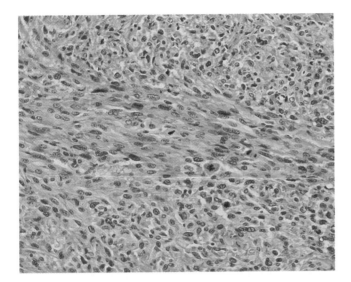

Fig. 10-58 Slightly angulated, fusiform nuclei with mitotic figures and irregularly distributed chromatin are seen in this malignant peripheral nerve sheath tumor.

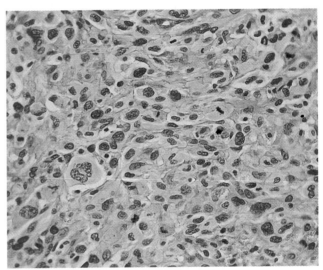

Fig. 10-59 Pleomorphic areas in a malignant peripheral nerve sheath tumor in which the cells have a histiocytoid appearance.

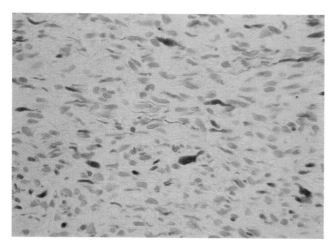

Fig. 10-60 S100 protein immunostaining is seen in 50% to 75% of malignant peripheral nerve sheath tumors.

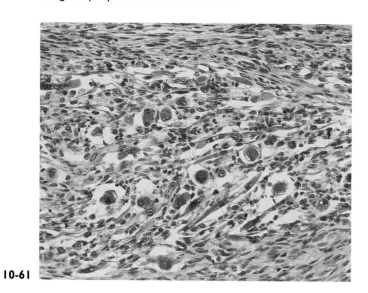

10-61

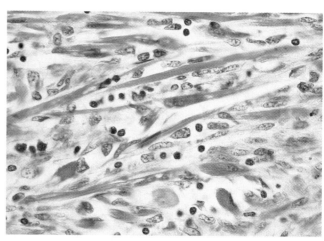

10-62

Figs. 10-61 and 10-62 Malignant Triton tumors with rhabdomyoblasts scattered amid relatively uniform primitive spindle cells.

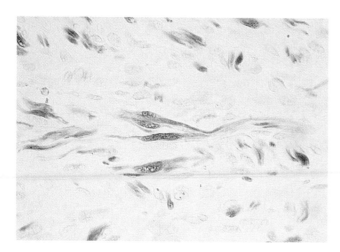

Fig. 10-63 S100 protein immunostaining in a malignant Triton tumor.

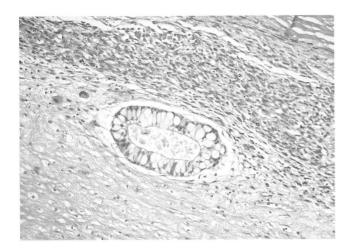

Fig. 10-64 Example of malignant peripheral nerve sheath tumor with gland formation. Mucin production may or may not be seen; the glands may be either benign or malignant. Glandular differentiation is much more common than squamous differentiation.

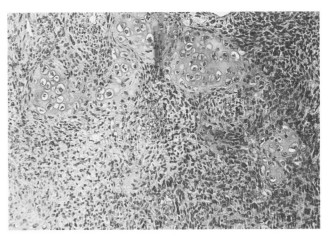

Fig. 10-65 Malignant peripheral nerve sheath tumor with cartilage formation. The cartilage is cytologically malignant, although this is not always the case.

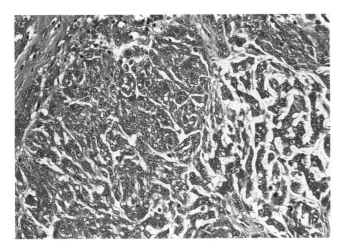

Fig. 10-66 An epithelioid malignant schwannoma in which plump, epithelioid cells are arranged in nests and cords with a background myxoid matrix.

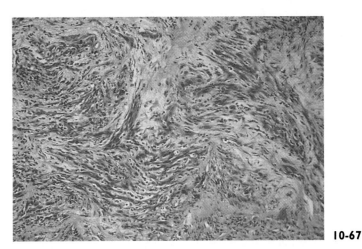

10-67

Figs. 10-67 through 10-71 Various examples of desmoplastic melanoma demonstrating a distinct neural appearance and associated with variable amounts of fibrosis and inflammation.

(Figs continued on next page.)

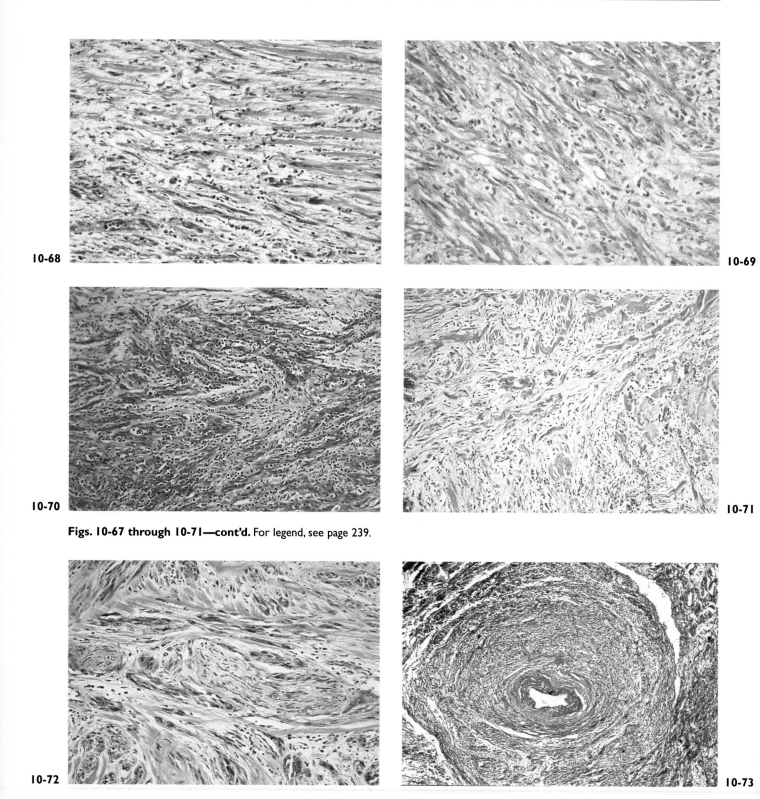

10-68

10-69

10-70

10-71

Figs. 10-67 through 10-71—cont'd. For legend, see page 239.

10-72

10-73

Figs. 10-72 and 10-73 A distinct association with a peripheral nerve may be seen in desmoplastic melanoma in addition to an angiocentric growth pattern (trichrome stains).

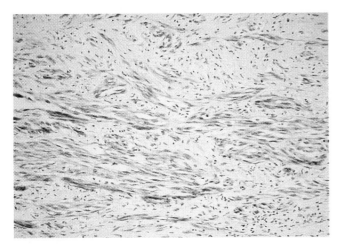

Fig. 10-74 Immunostains for S100 protein are usually positive, whereas staining for HMB45 is frequently negative in desmoplastic melanoma (S100 protein immunostain).

Malignant Granular Cell Tumor

Only 1% to 2% of granular cell tumors are estimated to be malignant. The clinical features of malignant granular cell tumor are, for the most part, similar to their benign counterparts. As mentioned previously, the histologic criteria are neither well defined nor absolute, but the following features are suggestive of potentially malignant behavior: (1) tumor size larger than 4 to 5 cm; (2) local recurrences, usually preceding metastases; (3) rapid growth; (4) more than 2 mitoses/10 hpf; (5) necrosis; (6) spindling of granular cells; (7) increased nuclear/cytoplasmic ratio; (8) hyperchromatic nuclei; and (9) distant metastases. Metastases occur most often to regional lymph nodes, followed by lung, liver, and bone.

MICROSCOPIC FEATURES

- See discussion of Malignant Granular Cell Tumor, Microscopic Features of Benign Granular Cell Tumor and Figures (pages 226-229).

DIFFERENTIAL DIAGNOSIS

- Benign granular cell tumor
- Leiomyosarcoma with granular cell change
- Angiosarcoma with granular cell change
- Alveolar soft part sarcoma
- Rhabdomyosarcoma
- Melanoma

242

Clear Cell Sarcoma (Malignant Melanoma Of Soft Parts)

Clear cell sarcoma is a distinctive sarcoma intimately associated with tendons and aponeuroses and possessing melanocytic features. Because of its melanocytic nature, it is believed to be derived from the neural crest. It typically occurs in the third and fourth decades of life, with a peak incidence in the third decade, and tends to affect the sexes equally. It has a proclivity to involve the deep tendinous structures of the distal extremities, particularly the foot and ankle. Patients present with a slowly growing mass that may be painful. Local recurrences, sometimes multiple, are not uncommon and may precede distant metastases; the latter are frequently to lungs, lymph nodes, bone, and occasionally the heart. Median intervals to local recurrences and metastases range from 2 to 3 years. Adverse prognostic factors are vascular invasion, presence of tumor necrosis, and larger tumor size. Metastases are almost invariably lethal. Prognosis remains poor despite adjuvant therapy.

MICROSCOPIC FEATURES

- Packeted arrangement of cells by delicate fibrous septa
- Fascicles simulating fibrosarcoma
- Uniform cells with clear to eosinophilic cytoplasm
- Abundant cytoplasmic glycogen
- Uniform round to oval nuclei with vesicular chromatin
- Prominent, large, basophilic nucleoli
- Multinucleated giant cells with uniform, peripherally oriented nuclei (wreath-like arrangement)
- Melanin (frequently inconspicuous)
- Hemosiderin
- Fibrosis (variable)

DIFFERENTIAL DIAGNOSIS

- Fibrosarcoma
- Malignant epithelioid schwannoma
- Acral lentiginous melanoma
- Desmoplastic and balloon cell melanoma
- Synovial sarcoma
- Renal cell carcinoma

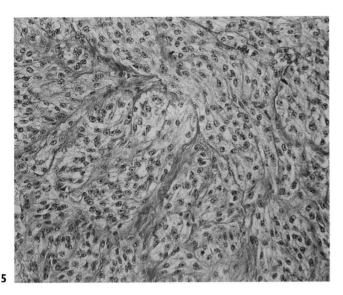

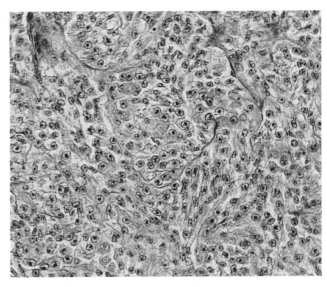

Figs. 10-75 and 10-76 Examples of clear cell sarcoma. Even at low magnification, a distinctive packeted to nested arrangement of cells can be seen in addition to an intimate association with the tendons and aponeuroses. A fascicular architecture may also be seen. The constituent cells range from round to oval to spindled. Typically at least some cells have prominent basophilic nucleoli, vesicular nuclei, and eosinophilic to clear cytoplasm.

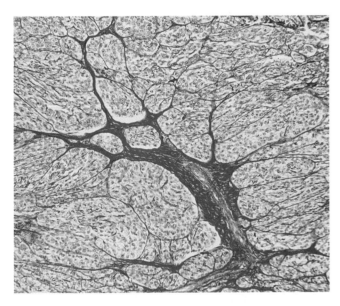

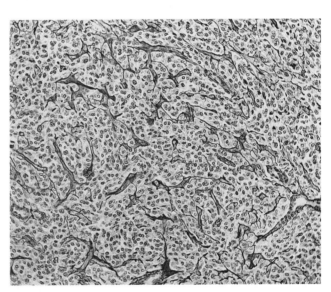

Fig. 10-77 A PAS stain with diastase digestion highlights the fibrous septa in clear cell sarcoma.

Fig. 10-78 Reticulin stains also highlight the nested arrangement of cells in clear cell sarcoma.

Malignant Melanotic Schwannoma

The criteria for malignancy in melanocytic schwannoma, as well as its psammomatous variant (other than distant metastases), are not well defined. Three histologic features have been described in psammomatous melanic schwanno-ma that have metastasized, although they are not unique to metastasizing lesions: (1) necrosis; (2) enlarged, pale nuclei with prominent, large, eosinophilic or violaceous nucleoli; and (3) numerous mitoses (see Benign Melanocytic Schwannoma—Microscopic Features and Differential Diagnosis).

Neuroblastoma and Ganglioneuroblastoma

Neuroblastoma and its maturing form, ganglioneuroblastoma, are primitive neuroectodermal tumors derived from the neural crest. They are one of the most common malignancies in childhood; one fourth are congenital and more than 500 new cases are diagnosed each year in the United States. Neuroblastoma arises along the sympathetic chain of nerves, occurring most frequently in the adrenal medulla; other locations include the neck, mediastinum, and retroperitoneum (primarily the organ of Zuckerkandl). It typically disseminates to bone marrow, bone, lymph nodes, and skin, and less frequently, to the dura mater and leptomeninges. The majority of cases are associated with elevated catecholamine levels or their metabolites. Patient age and clinical stage are important prognostic factors.

Nonadvanced disease (Evans stages I and II) tends to occur in children less than 1 year of age and generally responds to therapy. In contrast, advanced disease with or without distant metastases (Evans stages III and IV) tends to occur in older children and does not respond well to therapy. Histologic classification (Shimada et al.) is also of prognostic significance and in general reflects an age-matched maturational sequence, from neuroblastoma to ganglioneuroblastoma to ganglioneuroma, that may occur spontaneously. Amplification of N-*myc* is associated with a poor prognosis, although, paradoxically, aneuploid and hyperdipolid lesions have a better prognosis. Approximately 20% of neuroblastomas are related to a germline mutation, which is transmitted in an autosomal dominant manner. The most consistent chromosomal abnormality in neuroblastoma is the partial deletion of the short arm of chromosome 1.

MICROSCOPIC FEATURES

- Lobular or sheetlike growth pattern
- Thin fibrovascular septa
- Densely cellular to hypocellular
- Mats of neuropil/neurofibrillary stroma
- Primitive neuroblasts, 7 to 10 µm in diameter
- Dense, hyperchromatic nuclei
- Sparse cytoplasm
- Pseudorosettes
- True rosettes (rare)
- Mitoses and pyknotic (karyorrhectic) nuclei
- Crush artefact
- Calcification (variable)
- Maturation of neuroblasts to ganglion cells with: eosinophilic cytoplasm, vesicular chromatin, large nucleoli, and binucleate forms
- Maturation of stroma toward schwannian elements with a neurofibromatous appearance

DIFFERENTIAL DIAGNOSIS

- Ewing's sarcoma
- Lymphoma
- Granulocytic sarcoma
- Rhabdomyosarcoma
- Peripheral neuroepithelioma
- Neuroendocrine carcinoma of pulmonary or cutaneous origin
- Ganglioneuroma
- Pigmented neuroectodermal tumor of infancy
- Ectomesenchymoma

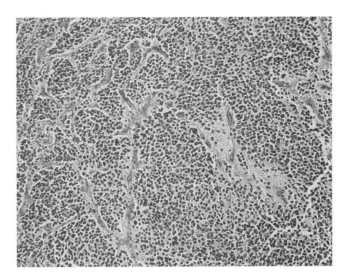

Fig. 10-79 Some small, rounded to angulated hyperchromatic cells associated with a variable amount of neuropil as well as compartmentalization by fibrous septa may be seen in neuroblastoma. The amount of hemorrhage and necrosis is variable.

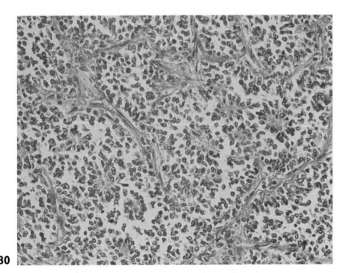

10-80

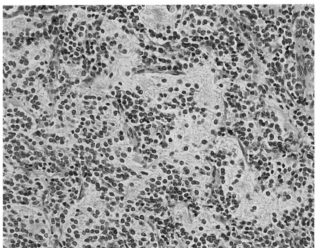

10-81

Figs. 10-80 through 10-82 Pseudorosettes are frequently seen in neuroblastoma and are attributable to the presence of centrally oriented neuropil surrounded by peripherally oriented nuclei of the neuroblasts.

10-82

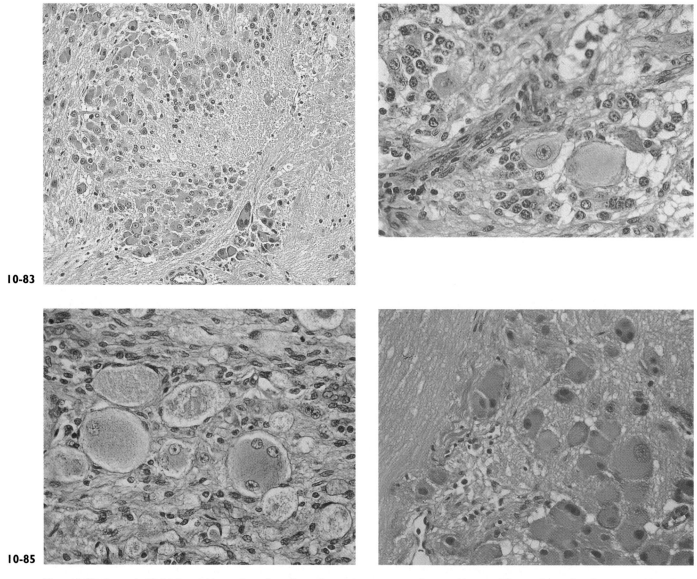

10-83

10-84

10-85

10-86

Figs. 10-83 through 10-86 A variable number of ganglion cells may be seen in ganglioneuroblastoma. The ganglion cell is characterized by a large vesicular nucleus with a prominent inclusion-like nucleolus and abundant amphophilic to eosinophilic cytoplasm. Scattered immature neuroblasts remain (Figs. 10-83 and 10-84). The matrix may be immature (neuropil) or exhibit schwannian maturation reminiscent of a neurofibroma.

Primitive Neuroectodermal Tumor (PNET)/Peripheral Neuroepithelioma

PNET/peripheral neuroeithelioma has also been referred to as peripheral neuroblastoma. Like neuroblastoma, it is a primitive proliferation of neural crest–derived cells with a capacity to differentiate toward neuronal and possibly schwannian structures. Unlike neuroblastoma, it occurs in a slightly older patient population, in a different location, and in general is far more aggressive. The majority of patients are adolescents or young adults. Approximately 60% occur in the limbs and limb girdles; many of those in the chest wall have been formerly referred to as Askin tumors. About one third of cases are associated with major peripheral nerve trunks, although there is no known association with von Recklinghausen's disease. This aggressive lesion tends to metastasize to lungs and lymph nodes. A reciprocal translocation of chromosomes 11 and 21, as well as tissue culture studies demonstrating a capacity for neuronal differentiation and expression of c-*myc*, suggest a close homology or relationship between PNET/peripheral neuroepithelioma and Ewing's sarcoma of bone.

MICROSCOPIC FEATURES

- Sheets or lobules of cells
- Primitive, small cells
- Scant cytoplasm
- Cytoplasmic glycogen
- Round to oval hyperchromatic nuclei
- Pseudorosettes (variable)

DIFFERENTIAL DIAGNOSIS

- Neuroblastoma
- Ewing's sarcoma, skeletal and extraskeletal
- Rhabdomyosarcoma
- Lymphoma
- Granulocytic sarcoma
- Neuroendocrine carcinoma of pulmonary or cutaneous origin

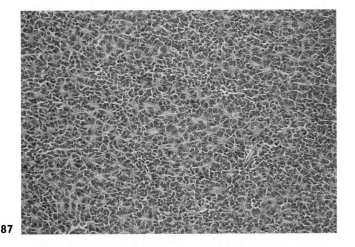
10-87

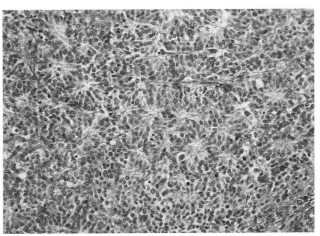
10-88

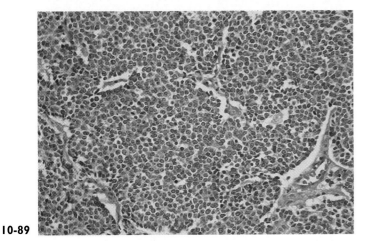
10-89

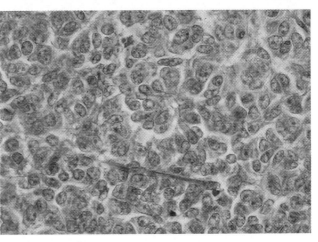
10-90

Figs. 10-87 through 10-90 Various examples of PNET/peripheral neuroepithelioma. Sheets of round, primitive cells with scant cytoplasm, a relatively homogeneous chromatin pattern, and small nucleoli are characterstic features. Intracytoplasmic glycogen is a variable finding. Pseudorosettes (Figs. 10-87 and 10-88) are frequently seen in peripheral neuroepithelioma but are not a prerequisite for the diagnosis.

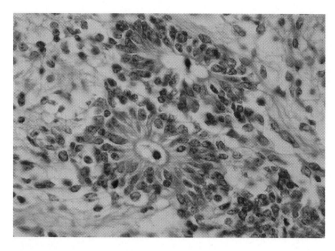

Fig. 10-91 True rosettes as seen here are very rare in neuro-epitheliomas.

Ectopic Ependymoma

True extraspinal ependymomas are rare and in general considered to be low-grade malignant neoplasms. They arise as slowly growing masses in the subcutis dorsal to the sacrococcygeal area and are most likely neural tube vestiges. Some are associated with spina bifida. Metastases tend to occur late and are to regional lymph nodes and lung.

MICROSCOPIC FEATURES

- Encapsulated
- Papillary configuration
- Fibrovascular stalks with prominent perivascular fibromyxoid zones
- Cuboidal to columnar ependymal cells
- Apically oriented nuclei
- Perivascular pseudorosettes
- Blepharoplasts (variable)

DIFFERENTIAL DIAGNOSIS

- Myxopapillary ependymoma of cauda equina
- Choroid plexus papilloma
- Extraskeletal myxoid chondrosarcoma
- Chordoma

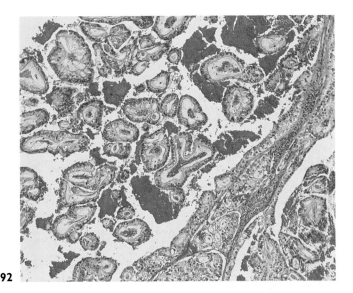

10-92

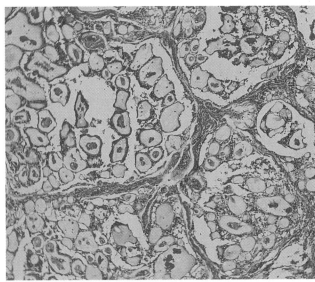

10-93

10-94

Figs. 10-92 through 10-94 Various examples of myxopapillary ependymoma, a lesion that arises in the differential diagnosis of ectopic or true extraspinal ependymoma. Extensive mucin deposition is seen in the connective tissue of the lesions' papillary fibrovascular cores (Fig. 10-94, colloidal iron stain). The ependymal cells range from cuboidal to columnar and have apically oriented nuclei.

Malignant Pigmented Neuroectodermal Tumor of Infancy

(See Benign Pigmented Neuroectodermal Tumor of Infancy—Discussion, Microscopic Features, Differential Diagnosis, and Figures, p. 233.)

Ectomesenchymoma

This extremely rare, malignant neoplasm occurs in children. It is unassociated with neurofibromatosis (von Recklinghausen's disease).

MICROSCOPIC FEATURES

- Mature ganglion cell elements
- Neurofibroma-like stroma

- Rhabdomyosarcomatous elements

DIFFERENTIAL DIAGNOSIS

- Ganglioneuroma
- Ganglioneuroblastoma
- Rhabdomyosarcoma

- Malignant Triton tumor
- Malignant mesenchymoma

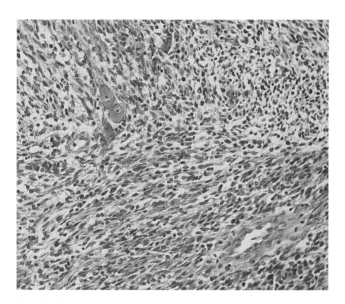

Fig. 10-95 An example of ectomesenchymoma illustrating ganglion cell elements in a background indistinguishable from malignant peripheral nerve sheath tumor or embryonal rhabdomyosarcoma.

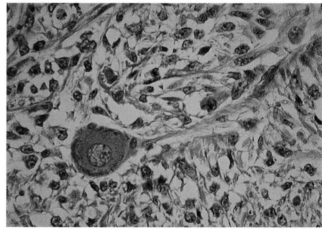

Fig. 10-96 Isolated ganglion cells intermingle with smaller rhabdomyoblasts with deeply acidophilic, elongated cytoplasmic processes in this case of ectomesenchymoma.

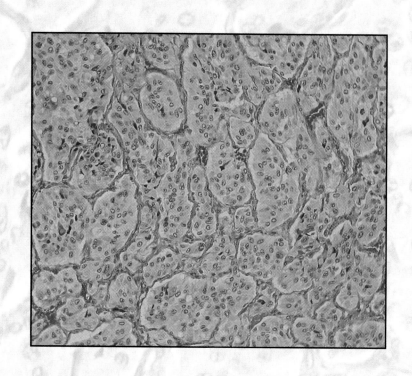

Chapter 11

Paraganglionic Tumors

BENIGN

Paraganglioma

Paragangliomas are unique neuroendocrine tumors of neural crest origin that arise in association with the autonomic ganglia. They are generally defined by their anatomic site and whether or not they are hormonally functional. Other than paragangliomas arising in the adrenal gland (pheochromocytoma), the most commonly occurring paragangliomas arise in the head and neck region (primarily carotid body, glomus jugulare, and vagal body paragangliomas) and the retroperitoneum (mainly in the organ of Zuckerkandl). Each paraganglioma has certain distinctive clinical features and varying degrees of aggressive biologic behavior.

The **carotid body paraganglioma,** which accounts for 60% of all head and neck paragangliomas, occurs more frequently in women at high altitudes, but otherwise has an equal sex distribution; 5% to 10% metastasize. In contrast, both the **glomus jugulare** and **vagal body paragangliomas** tend to occur in women; metastases are rare in the former, but may occur in 10% to 20% of cases in the latter. **Posterior mediastinal paragangliomas** and **retroperitoneal paragangliomas** are associated with the sympathetic chain and tend to display mixed histologic features of pheochromocytoma and carotid body paraganglioma. Ten to twenty percent of the retroperitoneal paragangliomas are extra-adrenal and 20% to 40% of them metastasize. The sex distribution is equal in this group, and most patients are between 30 and 45 years old.

Paragangliomas may be bilateral, hereditary, associated with paragangliomas at other body sites, or part of a variety of syndromes including Carney's triad and multiple endocrine neoplasia. As a rule, malignant paragangliomas metastasize to regional lymph nodes, and to a lesser extent, to the lungs, bone, and liver. Because the interval to metastasis may be long, extended follow-up is required. Clinical, macroscopic, and histologic criteria for malignancy in paraganglioma or any endocrine neoplasm are notoriously unreliable; extra-adrenal location, a multilobular configuration (grossly), mitoses, necrosis, pleomorphism, vascular invasion, a sheet-like pattern of growth, and absence of cytoplasmic hyaline globules are all reportedly suspicious features, but none of these alone is an absolute criterion or predictive of malignant behavior. The completeness of excision of the initial neoplasm correlates best with biologic behavior and eventual metastases; incompletely excised tumors tend to metastasize, whereas those that have been entirely removed do not. However, some types of paraganglioma, such as those arising in the glomus jugulare or aortic bodies of the anterior mediastinum, may be locally aggressive and cause significant morbidity and death.

MICROSCOPIC FEATURES

- Well circumscribed, partially encapsulated
- Extensive, delicate vascular network
- Nested groups of cells (zellballen)
- Syncytial arrangement of cells (variable)
- Ribbons and cords of cells
- Pseudoglandular or pseudorosette patterns
- Round to polygonal cells
- Pleomorphism (variable)
- Spindled cells (rare)
- Amphophilic to eosinophilic, granular cytoplasm
- Cytoplasmic vacuoles (pseudolipoblasts)
- Cytoplasmic hyaline globules (variable)
- Central, round nuclei
- Coarsely stippled chromatin
- Mitoses (variable)
- Marked sclerosis (variable)
- Hemorrhage (variable)
- Necrosis (variable)
- Ganglioneuromatous areas (variable)

DIFFERENTIAL DIAGNOSIS

- Gangliocytic paraganglioma
- Carcinoid
- Alveolar soft part sarcoma
- Carcinoma, adenocarcinoma
- Hemangiopericytoma
- Neuroblastoma
- Clear cell sarcoma

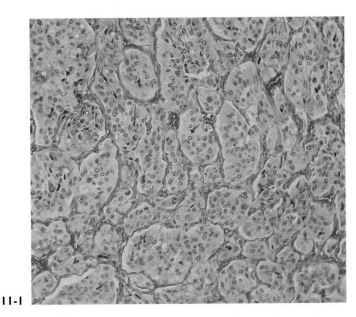

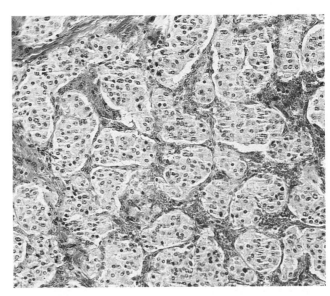

Figs. 11-1 and 11-2 Examples of paragangliomas demonstrating a nested pattern or arrangement of cells (zellballen) attributable to an underlying, delicate reticulin network and the occasional presence of prominent fibrous septa.

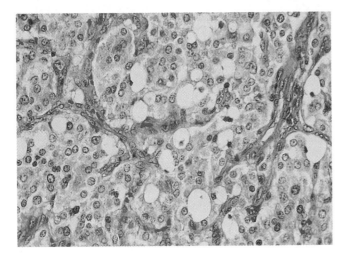

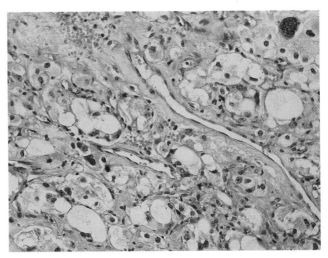

Fig. 11-3 Vacuolated cells with eosinophilic granular cytoplasm are a frequent feature of paraganglioma.

Fig. 11-4 Nuclear pleomorphism is not infrequent in paragangliomas, particularly in those occurring in the retroperitoneum. Some of those cases with multivacuolated clear cytoplasm and nuclear pleomorphism closely simulate lipoblasts.

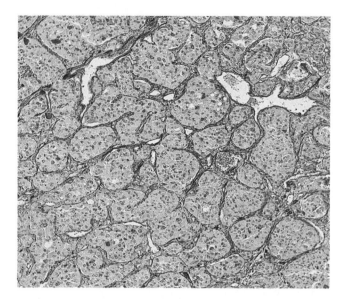

Fig. 11-5 The trichrome stain accentuates the nested architecture typical of paraganglioma.

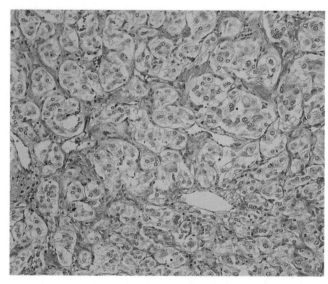

Fig. 11-6 Predominantly clear cells are seen in this example of pheochromocytoma.

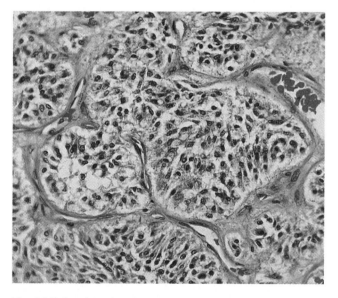

Fig. 11-7 Another pheochromocytoma with a prominent spindle cell pattern.

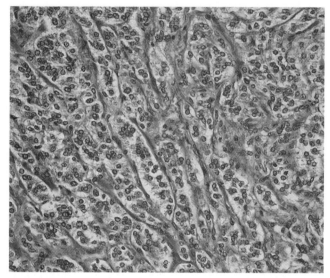

Fig. 11-8 A prominent cordlike pattern is seen in this pheochromocytoma.

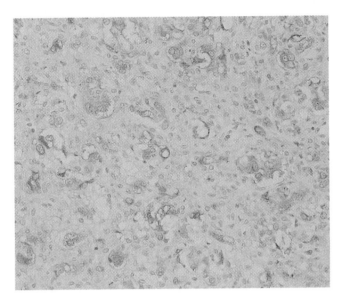

Fig. 11-9 Immunostains for chromogranin are seen in this pheochromocytoma.

MALIGNANT

Paraganglioma

The criteria to distinguish between benign and malignant paraganglioma are not well defined. Certain clinical, macroscopic, and histologic features, however, are suggestive of malignant potential (see Benign Paraganglioma—Discussion, Microscopic Features, and Differential Diagnosis, pp. 254-255).

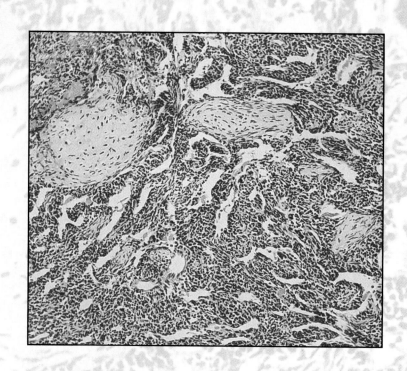

Chapter 12

Extraskeletal Osseous and Cartilaginous Tumors

BENIGN

Myositis Ossificans

This solitary, tender, self-limiting, reactive lesion is clearly related to trauma in approximately 50% of cases. It typically occurs in the musculature of the extremities of young, active men, especially the quadriceps and brachialis muscles. Occurrence in children is distinctly uncommon and should raise the question of fibrodysplasia ossificans progressiva. Nontraumatic cases may be seen in paraplegics or patients with a coagulopathy. Generally, a characteristic pattern of radiographic calcification is seen in lesions between 4 and 6 weeks after the initial insult; over time a shell of lamellar bone forms and changes to one which is heavily ossified, consisting solely of bone and fat with complete maturation. The latter remote lesions have been mistaken for osteomas. The radiographic stages of maturation seen in myositis ossificans correspond well with the microscopic features of a "zoning" phenomenon, wherein ossification proceeds from the periphery of the lesion toward the center. Lesions with similar microscopic features occur in the subcutis, fascia, and periosteum of the digits and are referred to as *panniculitis ossificans, fasciitis ossificans,* and *fibro-osseous pseudotumor of the digits,* respectively.

Panniculitis Ossificans

Approximately one third of cases with histologic features of myositis ossificans occur in the subcutis. In contrast to myositis ossificans, they tend to occur in the upper extremities of women. Age distribution and histology are similar to myositis ossificans, with the exception of a less prominent "zoning" phenomenon.

Fibro-osseous Pseudotumor of the Digits

This variant of myositis ossificans, also known as florid reactive periostitis of the digits, occurs primarily in the fingers and, to a lesser extent, the toes of young adults. In several cases there is a history of trauma, but unlike myositis ossificans, a "zoning" phenomeneon may not be apparent. There are occasional local recurrences. Radiographically, saucerization or erosion of the underlying cortical bone may be seen, similar to that seen in soft tissue or periosteal chondroma, as well as stippled calcifications.

Myositis Ossificans and its Variants

MICROSCOPIC FEATURES

- Well circumscribed
- "Zoning" phenomenon with maturation occurring first at periphery of lesion and proceeding centrally
- (Myo)fibroblastic core resembling nodular fasciitis (central)
- Osteoblasts
- Osteoclasts
- Chondrocytes (variable)
- Bland nuclear features
- Mild nuclear pleomorphism
- Mitoses
- Hemorrhage and hemorrhagic cysts or seromas (variable)
- Hemosiderin
- Multinucleated giant cells
- Inflammatory cells and fibrin
- Myxoid matrix (variable)
- Osteoid
- Lamellar bone
- Hyaline cartilage
- Endochondral calcification (variable)
- Entrapped, atrophic skeletal muscle fibers

DIFFERENTIAL DIAGNOSIS

- Nodular fasciitis
- Proliferative fasciitis and myositis
- Post-traumatic periostitis
- Fracture callus

- Fibrosdysplasia ossificans progressiva
- Fibrosarcoma
- Extraskeletal osteosarcoma

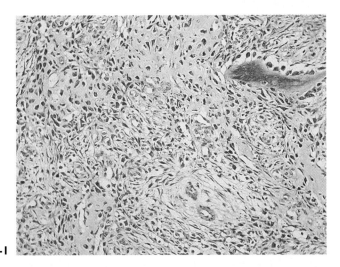

12-1

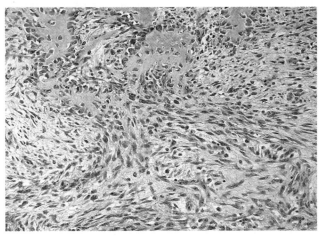

12-2

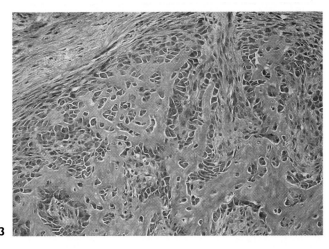

12-3

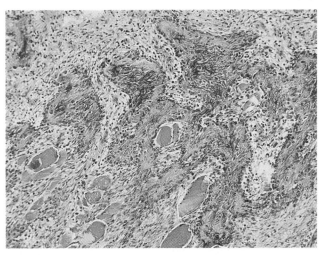

12-4

Figs. 12-1 through 12-6 Examples of myositis ossificans demonstrating bone formation amid a background cell population that is indistinguishable from nodular fasciitis. Numerous osteoblasts line islands of bone. Endochondral calcification may be seen (Figs. 12-5 and 12-6; colloidal iron stain, Fig. 12-6).

(Figs continued on next page.)

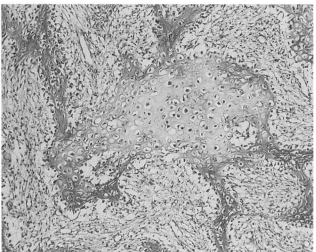

12-5

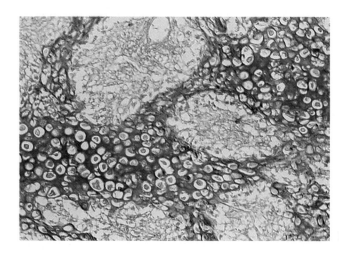

12-6

Figs. 12-1 through 12-6—cont'd. For legend, see page 261.

Fibrodysplasia (Myositis) Ossificans Progressiva

This slowly progressive, debilitating, hereditary disorder usually presents in children from infancy to 6 years of age, although older children and young adults may also be affected. It begins as a painful, soft tissue mass that involves skeletal muscle and the overlying subcutis. The paravertebral musculature, shoulders, occipital region, upper arms, and sternocleidomastoid muscle may be involved. With time, the soft tissue masses coalesce, fibrose, and calcify, leading to formation of "bony bridges" that cause restriction of respiration, ambulation, and deforming contractures. Digital malformations such as bilateral shortening of the fingers, absence of the thumbs and great toes, or bilateral hallux valgus, are also associated with the disease and, less frequently, exostoses, osteoporosis, sexual infantilism, and deafness. Although the disease course may be punctuated by remissions, it progresses slowly and within 10 to 15 years, many patients die from respiratory insufficiency. The underlying cause of the disease is not clear.

MICROSCOPIC FEATURES

- Ill defined and infiltrative
- Disorganized proliferaton of (myo)fibroblasts
- Interstitial edema
- Collagen (fibrosis)
- Skeletal muscle atrophy
- Irregular calcification/ossification without a "zoning" pattern
- Mature cartilage

DIFFERENTIAL DIAGNOSIS

- Infantile fibromatosis
- Proliferative fasciitis and myositis
- Myositis ossificans
- Nodular fasciitis
- Fracture calluses (battered child syndrome)
- Ectopic bone formation
- Pseudohypoparathyroidism

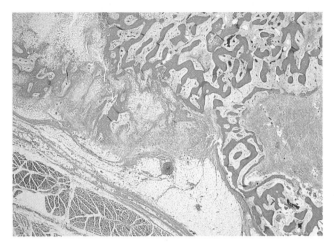

Fig. 12-7 Fibrodysplasia ossificans progressiva showing exclusive ossification of soft tissues.

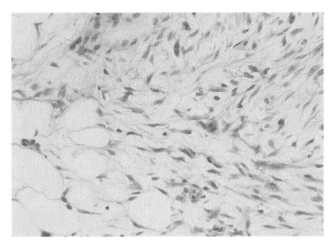

Fig. 12-8 Elongated, bland fibroblasts within a myxoid matrix infiltrate the adipose tissue in an early stage of fibrodysplasia ossificans progressiva.

Chondroma Of Soft Parts (Extraskeletal Chondroma)

Soft tissue chondroma occurs almost exclusively in the hands and the feet, primarily in adults in the fourth through sixth decades of life. It typically presents as a solitary, slowly enlarging mass of the fingers, which is by far the most common site. Lesions are frequently associated with tendons and may cause cortical erosion or saucerization of the underlying cortical bone, although they are not usually attached to the periosteum. Flocculent calcifications may be seen radiographically. Local recurrences are rare.

MICROSCOPIC FEATURES

- Well circumscribed
- Multinodular (variable)
- Relatively mature hyaline cartilage
- Hypercellular (variable)
- Immature or plump chondrocytes (variable)
- Nuclear atypia and binucleate cells (variable)
- Fibrous to myxoid matrix (variable)
- Epithelioid histiocytes (variable)
- Multinucleated giant cells (variable)
- Granular, flocculent, or punctate pattern of calcification (variable)

DIFFERENTIAL DIAGNOSIS

- Calcifying aponeurotic fibroma
- Tumoral calcinosis
- Giant cell tumor of tendon sheath (localized type)
- Subungual exostosis
- Subungual osteochondroma
- Periosteal chondroma
- Synovial chondromatosis
- Extraskeletal myxoid chondrosarcoma
- Well-differentiated chondrosarcoma
- Periosteal osteosarcoma

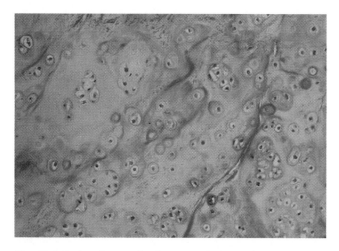

Fig. 12-9 A chondroma of soft parts with distinct hyaline cartilage formation.

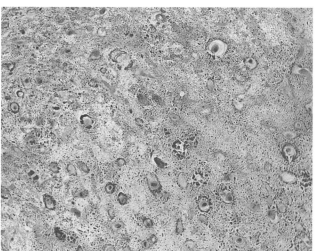

12-10A

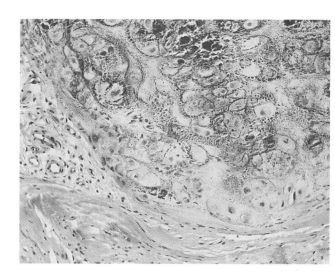

12-10B

Fig. 12-10 A and **B,** Examples of chondroma of soft parts with calcification.

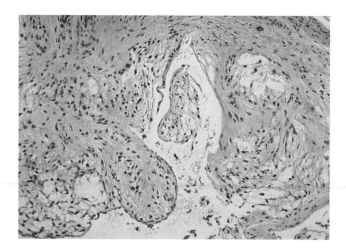

Fig. 12-11 Chondroma of soft parts with extensive myxoid change is frequently referred to as myxochondroma.

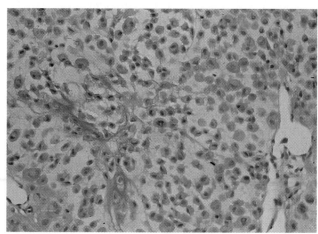

Fig. 12-12 A case of myxochondroma with plump epithelioid cells with abundant eosinophilic cytoplasm.

MALIGNANT

Extraskeletal Chondrosarcoma

Well-Differentiated Extraskeletal Chondrosarcoma

This extremely rare variant of chondrosarcoma may occur in soft tissue; well-differentiated chon-drosarcomas of bone are far more common and better characterized. Too few cases have been reported to draw conclusions or make generalizations. Cases of chondrosarcoma arising in synovial chondromatosis are not included in this category.

MICROSCOPIC FEATURES

- Well circumscribed
- Hypercellular, well-differentiated hyaline cartilage
- Mild nuclear atypia
- Binucleate chondrocytes
- Rare mitoses
- Calcification (variable)

DIFFERENTIAL DIAGNOSIS

- Chondroma of soft parts
- Osteochondroma
- Benign or malignant mesenchymoma with cartilage
- Chondrosarcoma arising in osteochondroma
- Well-differentiated chondrosarcoma of bone
- Periosteal osteosarcoma
- Malignant peripheral nerve sheath tumor with chondroid metaplasia

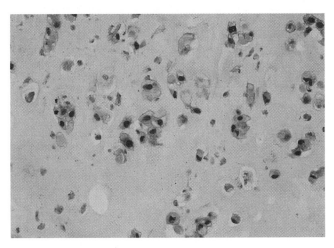

Fig. 12-13 Well-differentiated extraskeletal chondrosarcoma showing mild pleomorphism of the chondrocytes; some are binucleate.

Extraskeletal Myxoid Chondrosarcoma

This slowly growing, deep-seated mass typically occurs in the musculature of adults, with a median age of onset of 50 years. Men are affected approximately twice as often as women. The distal extremities and its limb girdles are involved in 70% of cases, followed by the trunk (20%) and the upper extremities and limb girdles (10%). It is a relatively low-grade sarcoma, in contrast to its counterpart in bone. Approximately 75% of patients are alive at 10 years, with a local recurrence rate of 50% to 55%, and metastases in 40% to 45% of patients at 10 years. Local recurrences are frequently multiple. Detection of metastases may precede or be found at the time of diagnosis in up to 40% of cases. Survival times of 5 to 15 years after the development of lung metastases are not uncommon. The most frequent sites of metastases are the lungs, followed by lymph nodes, bone, and brain. Large tumor size (especially >10 cm) and advanced age are poor prognostic factors.

MICROSCOPIC FEATURES

- Well circumscribed
- Fibrous capsule
- Multilobular with fibrous septa
- Abundant myxoid matrix (hyaluronidase resistant)
- Interanastomosing strands or filigreed arrangement of chondroblasts
- Small, round to oval to slender, elongated chondroblasts
- Scant, eosinophilic cytoplasm
- Glycogen (cytoplasmic)
- Hyperchromatic nuclei
- Mitoses (variable)
- Necrosis (variable)
- Hypercellular (rare)
- Hyaline cartilage (variable)
- Secondary changes including: hemorrhage, hemosiderin, fibrosis
- Calcification (rare)

DIFFERENTIAL DIAGNOSIS

- Myxoma
- Myxochondroma of soft parts
- Parachordoma
- Chordoma
- Chondromyxoid fibroma (soft tissue extension)
- Lipoma or its variants with extensive chondroid metaplasia
- Myxoid liposarcoma
- Periosteal osteosarcoma
- Myoepithelial neoplasms, including mixed tumors of skin and salivary gland
- Myxopapillary ependymoma
- Mixed tumor

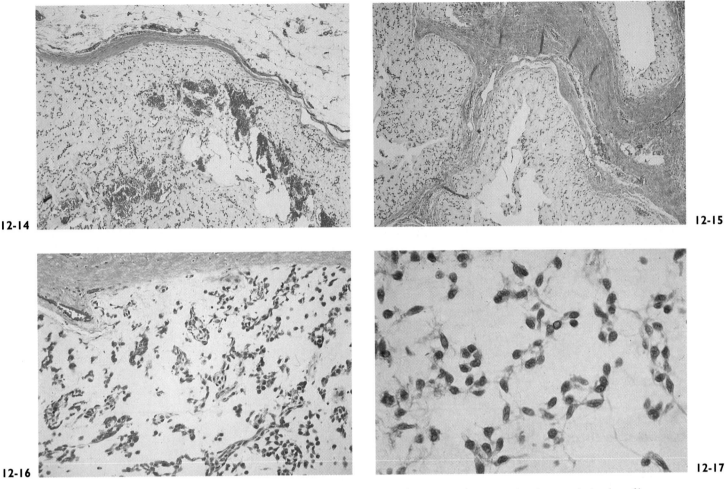

12-14

12-15

12-16

12-17

Figs. 12-14 through 12-17 Typical examples of extraskeletal myxoid chondrosarcoma demonstrating circumscription by a fibrous capsule, which extends into the lesion and divides it into multiple lobules. An abundant hypovascular myxoid matrix contains delicate strands and nests of immature chondrocytes with nuclei that are usually small and hyperchromatic.

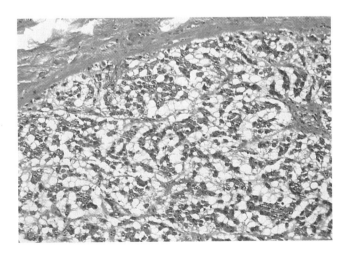

Fig. 12-18 A more cellular example of extraskeletal myxoid chondrosarcoma.

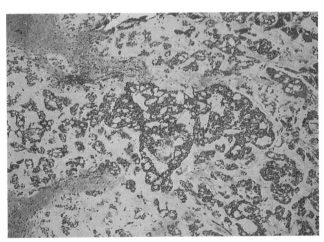

Fig. 12-19 Example of extraskeletal myxoid chondrosarcoma with a cribriform arrangement of cells.

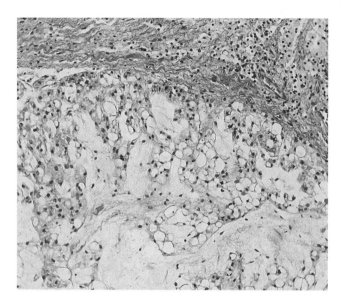

Fig. 12-20 Microscopic appearance of chordoma demonstrating nests and strands of glycogen-rich cells with clear, vacuolated cytoplasm (physaliferous cells) within an abundant myxoid matrix. Some of the cells have eosinophilic cytoplasm and range from polygonal to spindled in shape. Chordoma, especially its metastases, may be confused with extraskeletal myxoid chondrosarcoma and cutaneous mixed tumor.

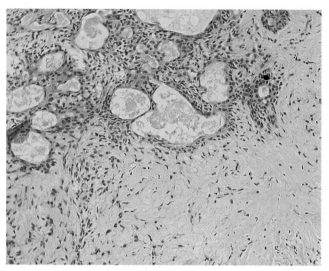

Fig. 12-21 Cutaneous mixed tumor with prominent myxoid zones. If the epithelial elements are inconspicuous and the myxoid matrix prominent, lesions may be easily mistaken for a myxoid chondrosarcoma.

Extraskeletal Mesenchymal Chondrosarcoma

This highly malignant neoplasm is more common in bone than in soft tissue. The soft tissue tumors have a bimodal age distribution related to anatomic location. Lesions of the head and neck region (particularly meningeal and periorbital tumors) tend to occur in patients around 25 years of age, whereas those that involve the deep musculature such as the thigh occur in patients approximately 45 years old. Men and women are affected equally. Symptoms are referable to a mass effect and include those associated with increased intracranial pressure or visual symptoms in the head and neck cases. Calcification may be detected radiographically. The clinical course is aggressive with frequent metastases, primarily to lungs and lymph nodes. Histologic features, such as the degree of chondroid differentiation, appear to have no bearing on prognosis.

MICROSCOPIC FEATURES

- Relatively well circumscribed
- Nodules of cartilage, dense collagen, or bone
- Relatively uniform, primitive, small, round to spindled cells
- Sheets of primitive undifferentiated cells
- Scant cytoplasm
- Hemangiopericytic vascular pattern
- Fibrosis (variable)

DIFFERENTIAL DIAGNOSIS

- Hemangiopericytoma
- Synovial sarcoma
- Localized fibrous tumor of pleura/peritoneum

- Ewing's sarcoma
- Peripheral neuroepithelioma

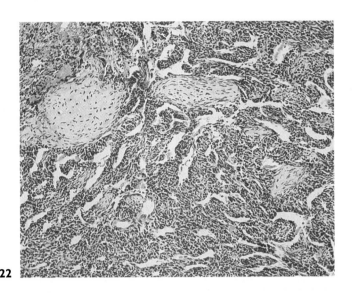

12-22

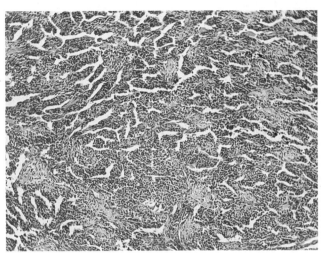

12-23

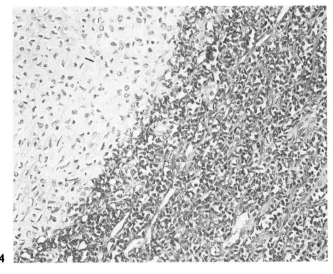

12-24

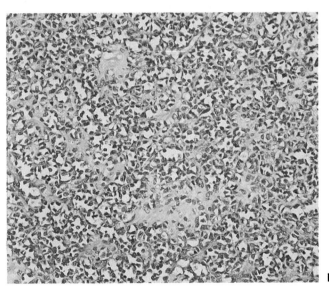

12-25

Figs. 12-22 through 12-25 Typical examples of extraskeletal mesenchymal chondrosarcoma demonstrating a prominent hemangiopericytic vascular pattern and scattered nodules of chondrohyaline matrix amid a population of small, primitive cells with hyperchromatic nuclei and scant cytoplasm.

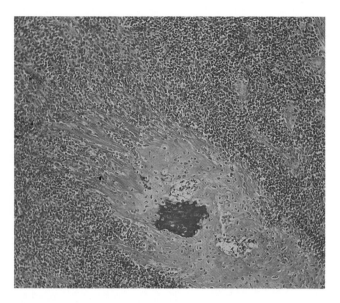

Fig. 12-26 Some of the chondrohyaline nodules of extraskeletal mesenchymal chondrosarcoma are focally calcified.

Extraskeletal Osteosarcoma

Extraskeletal osteosarcoma is a malignant neoplasm that forms osteoid and does not arise in bone. It is much rarer than its osseous counterpart and accounts for less than 5% of all osteosarcomas. It also arises in an older patient population than conventional osteosarcoma of bone, generally afflicting patients 45 to 55 years of age. Some cases are radiation induced, following treatment for other malignant neoplasms such as Hodgkin's disease, carcinoma of the breast or female genital tract, and retinoblastoma. Others have been associated with a prior history of Thorotrast administration. Typically, it presents as a deep-seated mass,

frequently in the thigh or retroperitoneum, and is associated with pain in up to one third of cases. The microscopic features generally reflect those of the histologic subtypes that have been delineated in skeletal osteosarcomas, including fibroblastic, osteoblastic, chondroblastic, and less commonly telangiectatic types of osteosarcoma. The small cell variant of osteosarcoma, however, is unusual. The prognosis is grim; 50% to 75% of patients are dead of disease within a few years despite radical surgery and adjuvant therapy. Metastases are usually to lungs and lymph nodes. Patients with tumors larger than 5 cm fare worse than those with smaller tumors.

MICROSCOPIC FEATURES

- Circumscribed or ill defined
- Osteoid elaborated by malignant cells
- Delicate, lacelike strands to trabecular or amorphous deposits of osteoid
- Hyaline cartilage (variable)
- Ossification or lamellar bone (variable)
- Malignant osteoblasts, fibroblasts, fibrohistiocytic cells, and chondrocytes
- Pleomorphic to bizarre cells
- Mitoses
- Multinucleated giant cells, benign or malignant (variable)
- Osteoclast-like giant cells
- Aneurysmal, hemorrhagic foci (variable)
- Areas resembling fibrosarcoma, malignant fibrous histiocytoma, chondrosarcoma, or a "round cell" (small cell) pattern

DIFFERENTIAL DIAGNOSIS

- Carcinosarcoma
- Malignant mesenchymoma
- Malignant fibrous histiocytoma (especially with osteoid)
- Synovial sarcoma with metaplastic bone
- Epithelioid sarcoma with metaplastic bone
- Liposarcoma with metaplastic bone

- Conventional osteosarcoma of bone
- High-grade surface osteosarcoma
- Parosteal osteosarcoma
- Periosteal osteosarcoma
- Conventional chondrosarcoma of bone with ossification

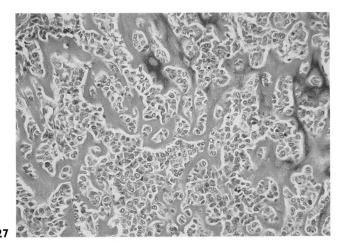

12-27

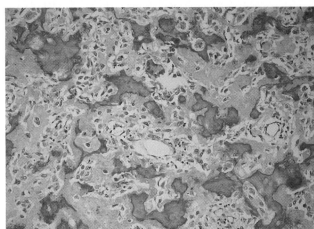

12-28

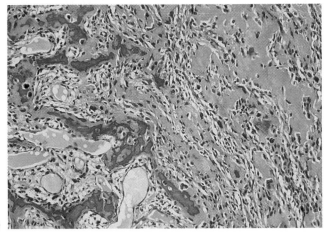

12-29

Figs. 12-27 through 12-29 Cases of extraskeletal osteosarcoma demonstrating calcified bone trabeculae, osteoid and osteoid that is becoming calcified.

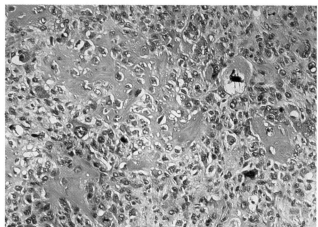

12-30

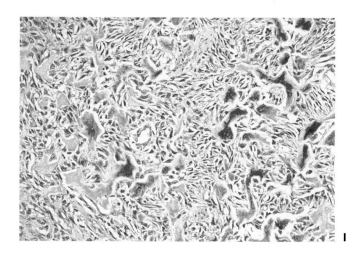

12-31

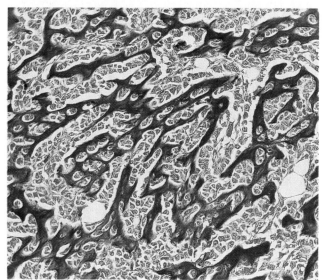

12-32

Figs. 12-30 through 12-32 Additional examples of extraskeletal osteosarcoma demonstrating a variety of appearances of the malignant cell population as well as extracellular matrix production. Fig. 12-31 is a postradiation osteosarcoma. (Fig. 12-32, trichrome stain).

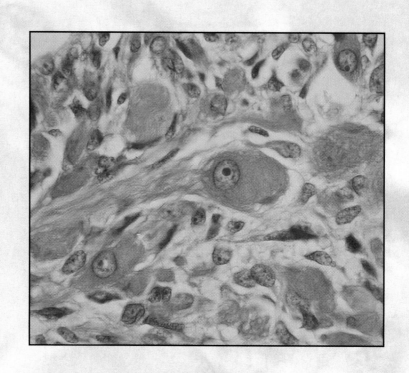

Chapter 13

Pluripotential Mesenchymal Tumors

BENIGN

Benign Mesenchymoma

Benign mesenchymoma is a lesion of soft tissue that contains two or more well-defined or differentiated components. Examples include lipomas with chondroid or osseous metaplasia, myolipoma of soft tissue, and benign Triton tumor. Intramuscular hemangiomas have been confused with benign mesenchymomas because of the presence of fatty overgrowth, which is not an intrinsic part of the neoplasm. In general the major component of benign mesenchymoma such as adipose tissue, dictates the clinical behavior, and the lesion is named according to the predominant component. The term *benign mesenchymoma* is rarely used because it conveys minimal information and refers to a diverse group of lesions.

MICROSCOPIC FEATURES

- See Microscopic Features of individual benign tumors

DIFFERENTIAL DIAGNOSIS

- See Differential Diagnosis of individual benign tumors

MALIGNANT

Malignant Mesenchymoma

Malignant mesenchymoma is a malignant mesenchymal neoplasm that displays the features of at least two distinct and unrelated sarcomas, excluding fibrosarcoma, malignant fibrous histiocytoma, and hemangiopericytoma. This heterogeneous group of tumors tends to occur in the retroperitoneum and thigh of adults beyond the fifth decade of life. The nomenclature and prognosis of these tumors are usually dictated by the predominant histologic component. Common combinations of sarcoma include liposarcoma with rhabdomyosarcoma, leiomyosarcoma, or osteosarcoma. Certain types of neoplasms such as liposarcoma and malignant peripheral nerve sheath tumor sometimes display chondroid or osseous differentiation, which may or may not appear to be histologically malignant. These tumors are generally not referred to as malignant mesenchymomas. Moreover, well-defined tumors such as malignant Triton tumor and ectomesenchymoma are technically malignant mesenchymomas but are usually not referred to as such. Malignant mesenchymomas presumably arise from primitive mesenchymal cells that possess the capacity to differentiate along multiple pathways.

MICROSCOPIC FEATURES

- See Microscopic Features of individual types of sarcomas

DIFFERENTIAL DIAGNOSIS

- Immature teratoma with sarcomatous overgrowth
- Cystosarcoma phyllodes with sarcomatous overgrowth
- Adenosarcoma with sarcomatous overgrowth
- Metaplastic breast carcinoma
- Malignant mixed müllerian tumor
- Carcinosarcoma
- Sarcomatoid carcinoma
- Collision tumor

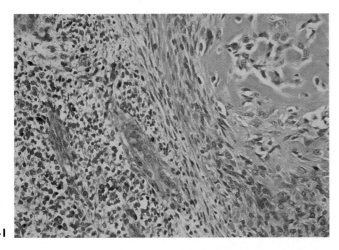
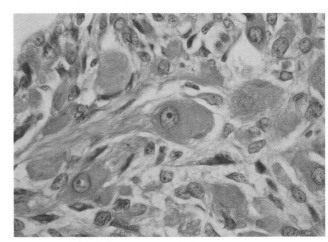

13-1   13-2

Figs. 13-1 and 13-2 Osteosteosarcoma (Fig. 13-1) and rhabdomyosarcoma (Fig. 13-2) in different portions of this malignant mesenchymoma.

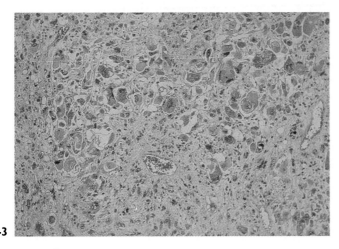
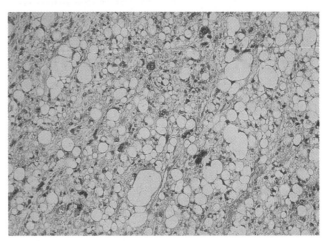

13-3   13-4

Figs. 13-3 and 13-4 Malignant mesenchymoma demonstrating rhabdomyosarcomatous (Fig. 13-3) and liposarcomatous (Fig. 13-4) elements.

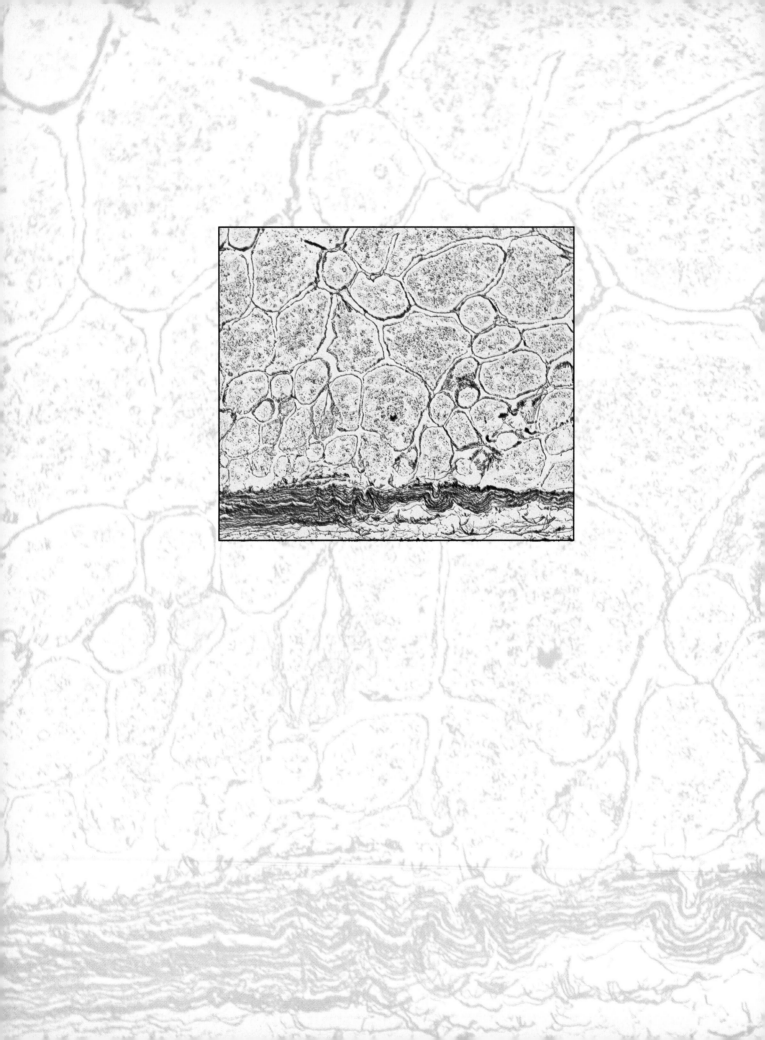

Chapter 14

Tumors of Uncertain Histogenesis

BENIGN

Congenital Granular Cell Tumor

This unusual proliferation of granular cells occurs exclusively along the upper alveolar ridge of the jaw in infants. Approximately 10% of lesions are multiple, and the majority of patients are girls. Spontaneous regression is not uncommon. Although it bears a close histologic similarity to granular cell tumor of neural origin, the tumor does not stain for S100 protein; moreover, ultrastructural studies display cells with histiocytic and fibroblastic features containing fat and lysosomes.

MICROSCOPIC FEATURES

- See Benign Granular Cell Tumor
- Prominent vascularity

- Scattered odontogenic remnants

DIFFERENTIAL DIAGNOSIS

- Granular cell tumor

- Fibrous histiocytoma

Tumoral Calcinosis

Tumoral calcinosis is an idiopathic disorder characterized by the presence of large calcified nodules in the periarticular soft tissues around large joints such as the greater trochanter, gluteal region, shoulder, and elbow. It typically presents in the first two decades of life, is slightly more common in males than females, affects siblings in 50% and black patients in two thirds of cases, and is unassociated with other conditions such as chronic renal failure with secondary hyperparathyroidism or collagen vascular disease. Serum phosphate levels are usually elevated, but the calcium level is normal. Smaller lesions are amenable to complete surgical excision; in contrast, larger lesions may ulcerate the skin or become infected.

MICROSCOPIC FEATURES

- Unencapsulated, but relatively well defined
- Multinodular
- Fibrous septa
- Multinucleated giant cells, osteoclast-like giant cells, and macrophages surrounding calcified areas ("active" lesions)

- Central zones of granular, amorphous, calcified material
- Dense, fibrous connective tissue surrounding calcified material ("inactive" lesions)
- Psammomatous calcifications (rare)

DIFFERENTIAL DIAGNOSIS

- Chronic renal failure with secondary hyperparathyroidism
- Hypervitaminosis D
- Milk alkali syndrome
- Osteolysis secondary to neoplasia or infection

- Dystrophic calcifications from various conditions
- Calcinosis cutis associated with collagen vascular/ autoimmune diseases
- Amyloidoma

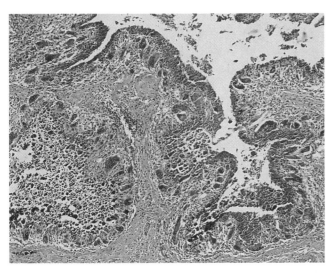

Fig. 14-1 A case of tumoral calcinosis showing cyst-like spaces lined by dense fibrous connective tissue, multinucleated giant cells, and macrophages and associated with granular calcified material.

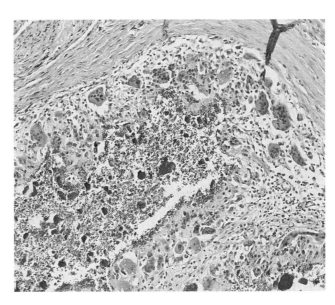

14-2

Figs. 14-2 through 14-4 Additional examples of tumoral calcinosis demonstrating a variable number of multinucleated giant cells, fibrosis, and calcification. Concentric calcifications with a psammomatous appearance are unusual.

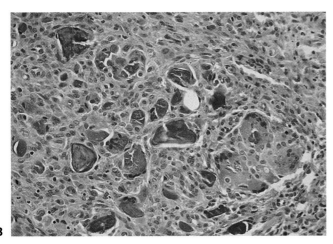

14-3

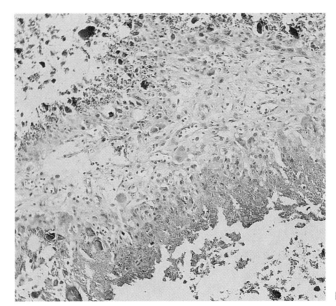

14-4

Myxoma

Myxomas are localized growths of fibroblast-like cells in an abundant myxoid matrix. Whether they are reactive or neoplastic is unclear. The three main variants of myxoma are the intramuscular, cutaneous, and juxta-articular types. Although they share several histologic features, they occur in distinctive clinical settings.

Intramuscular Myxoma

This tumor usually presents in the fifth through seventh decades of life and tends to occur in the large muscles of the body, particulary the thigh, buttock, shoulder, and upper arm. The lesions may be entirely intramuscular or associated with skeletal muscle fascia. Symptoms are usually referable to a mass. Occasional cases (multiple myxomas) may be associated with fibrous dysplasia and conditions such as Albright's syndrome and hypophosphatemic osteomalacia. Local recurrences are rare despite incomplete excision.

Cutaneous Myxoma

Myxomas occurring in the subcutis may be sporadic or associated with Carney's complex, which is transmitted as an autosomal dominant trait and associated with cardiac myxomas, spotty pigmenta-tion, endocrine overactivity, and psammomatous melanotic schwannomas. The percentage of myxomas unassociated with the complex is not known; the majority are probably not associated with it. Histologically, cutaneous myxomas are similar to their intramuscular counterpart, except that they are often not as well demarcated or multilobulated.

Juxta-articular Myxoma

This periarticular variant of myxoma is frequently associated with cysts. Approximately 90% of cases occur in the region of the knee, with one fourth involving the meniscus. The remainder tend to occur around large joints such as the shoulder, elbow, hip, and ankle, although the wrist and the hand may rarely be involved. Approximately 90% of juxta-articular myxomas (JAM) contain cysts that closely resemble ganglions. Most cases occur in men (75%) in the third through seventh decades of life. Frequently, there is evidence of associated degenerative joint disease. This particular variant of myxoma is unique because it may involve the subcutis, periarticular dense fibrous connective tissues, and the joint itself (meniscus and synovium) and it is not associated with other syndromes or tumors. Local recurrences, sometimes multiple, are not uncommon.

Intramuscular, Cutaneous, and Juxta-articular Myxomas

MICROSCOPIC FEATURES

- Well circumscribed to ill defined
- Vague multinodular to diffuse pattern (cutaneous myxoma and JAM)
- Incomplete fibrous septa
- Abundant myxoid stroma
- Hypovascular
- Paucicellular
- Scattered macrophages containing lipid or mucin (variable)

- Bland, fibroblast-like cells, spindled to stellate
- Atrophic skeletal muscle fibers (intramuscular myxoma and JAM)
- Entrapped epithelial elements (cutaneous myxoma)
- Entrapped islets of fat (cutaneous myxoma and JAM)
- Cyst formation resembling a ganglion cyst (intramuscular myxoma and JAM)
- Fibrosis and hemorrhage (JAM)
- Reactive (myo)fibroblastic proliferation (JAM)

DIFFERENTIAL DIAGNOSIS

- Ganglion cyst
- Cutaneous myxoid cyst
- Dermal mucinoses, including localized myxedema
- Myxoid neurofibroma
- Myxoid neurothekeoma
- Nodular fasciitis
- Myxolipoma

- Myxochondroma
- Myxoid dermatofibrosarcoma protuberans
- Myxoid malignant fibrous histiocytoma
- Extraskeletal myxoid chondrosarcoma
- Myxoid liposarcoma
- Botryoid rhabdomyosarcoma

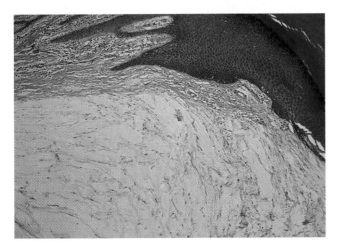

Fig. 14-5 Low magnification of a subungual myxoma showing a well-demarcated, hypocellular myxoid lesion in the dermis and subcutis.

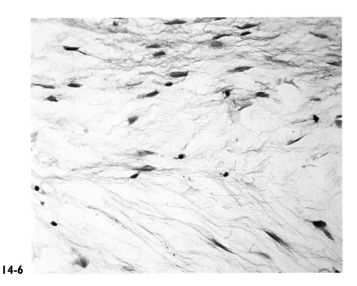

14-6

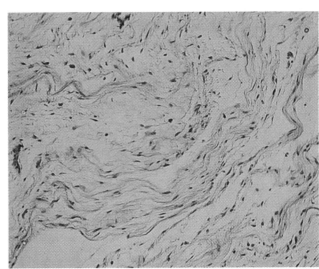

14-7

Figs. 14-6 through 14-9 Various examples of intramuscular myxoma showing a hypocellular lesion composed of cytologically bland cells resembling fibroblasts in an abundant and hypovascular myxoid matrix.

(Figs continued on next page.)

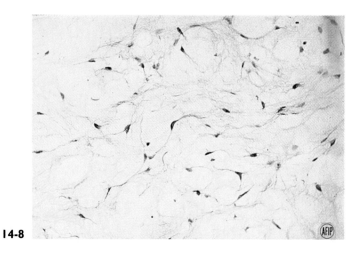

14-8

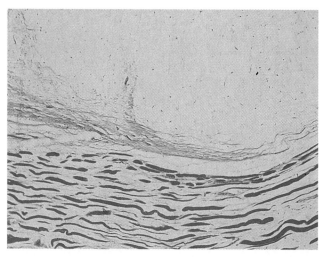

14-9

Figs. 14-6 through 14-9—cont'd. For legend, see page 283.

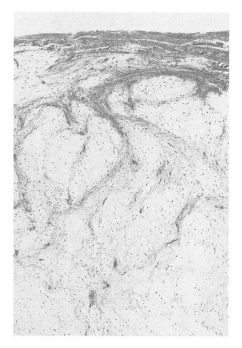

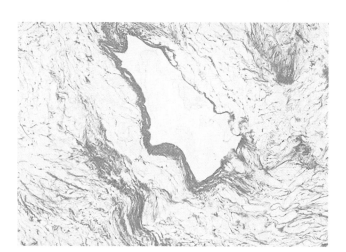

Fig. 14-11 Cysts with fibrotic walls of varying thickness, resembling ganglion cysts, are seen in most juxta-articular myxomas.

Fig. 14-10 Juxta-articular myxoma subjacent to synovium. Note incomplete fibrous septa, similar to those seen in intramuscular myxoma.

Angiomyxoma

This relatively rare lesion has been referred to in the literature as aggressive angiomyxoma. It typically occurs as a large, ill-defined soft tissue mass in the pelvis, perineum, or genital region in women, although rare cases have been reported in men. There is a high rate of local recurrence, but metastases have not been reported.

MICROSCOPIC FEATURES

- Ill-defined margins
- Prominent vasculature of small to medium caliber with thin and thick walls
- Abundant, myxoid matrix
- Spindled to stellate fibroblast-like cells
- Cytologically bland nuclei
- Few mitoses
- Variable fibrosis

DIFFERENTIAL DIAGNOSIS

- Myxoid neurofibroma
- Myxoma
- Myxolipoma
- Angiomyofibroblastoma
- Spindle cell lipoma
- Myxoid leiomyoma
- Myxoid leiomyosarcoma
- Myxoid malignant fibrous histiocytoma
- Myxoid liposarcoma
- Botryoid rhabdomyosarcoma

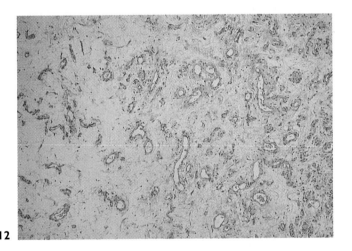

14-12

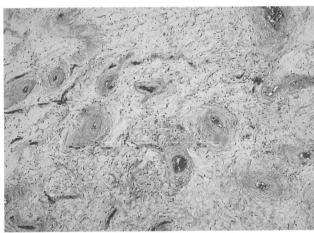

14-13

14-14

Figs. 14-12 through 14-14 Examples of angiomyxoma showing numerous vessels of varying thickness associated with a myxoid matrix. The trichrome stain (Fig. 14-14) accentuates the fibrotic areas, especially around some of the blood vessels.

Amyloidoma

Amyloidomas are relatively rare in soft tissue, although they have been described in a variety of other sites including the respiratory tract, gastrointestinal tract, urinary tract, skin, and joints. They may be either primary (unassociated with an underlying cause) or secondary (associated with myeloma, chronic infection, or chronic inflammation). Lesions may be either solitary or multiple.

MICROSCOPIC FEATURES

- Circumscribed
- Vaguely lobulated
- Amorphous eosinophilic material (metachromatic, Congophilic, and birefringent)
- Surrounded by multinucleated giant cells, plasma cells, and lymphocytes
- Blood vessels thicked by amyloid
- Cartilage and ossification (variable)

DIFFERENTIAL DIAGNOSIS

- Elastofibroma
- Tumoral calcinosis
- Hyalin fibromatosis

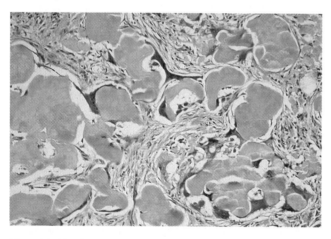

Fig. 14-15 Example of amyloid tumor with amorphous, eosinophilic material surrounded by multinucleated giant cells.

Parachordoma

This extraordinarily rare neoplasm of young adults occurs in the deep soft tissues of the extremities, usually in close proximity to tendons, synovium, or bone. They may recur, but metastases have not been reported.

MICROSCOPIC FEATURES

- Lobulated
- Nests or vaguely acinar arrangements of cells
- Polygonal to spindled cells
- Clear to vacuolated cytoplasm (glycogen)
- Vesicular or pyknotic nuclei
- Myxoid matrix (hyaluronidase sensitive)
- Hyalinization (variable)

DIFFERENTIAL DIAGNOSIS

- Mixed (myoepithelial) tumor of skin
- Chondroid lipoma
- Myxochondroma of soft parts
- Mixed tumor of adnexal origin (chondrosyringoma)

- Variant of liposarcoma
- Metastatic chordoma
- Extraskeletal myxoid chondrosarcoma

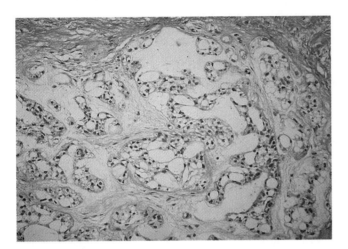

Fig. 14-16 Example of a parachordoma in which the cells with clear, glycogen-rich cytoplasm are arranged in nests and strands in an abundant myxoid matrix.

BORDERLINE

Ossifying Fibromyxoid Tumor of Soft Parts

Ossifying fibromyxoid tumor of soft parts (OFT) is a recently described lesion of probable neural derivation that typically occurs in the deep subcutis of adults, with a median age of onset of 50 years. It was originally described as being surrounded by an incomplete shell of lamellar bone (**ossifying**), but more recent evidence suggests that many lesions probably do not have a shell of bone (**nonossify-**

ing). OFT is a slowly growing, painless mass that primarily involves the extremities (70%), followed by the trunk (20%) and the head and neck (10%). Attachment to tendon, fascia, and skeletal muscle may occur; origin from a nerve trunk has not been documented. Approximately one third of cases recur locally; these may be multiple, particularly in cellular, mitotically active, deep, large, or cytologically malignant tumors. Evidence suggests that lesion is probably a unique peripheral nerve sheath tumor with a propensity for local recurrences, although metastases are distinctly rare.

MICROSCOPIC FEATURES

- Circumscribed
- Fibrous capsule
- Incomplete shell of lamellar bone (variable)
- Multinodular (variable)
- Fibrous septa
- Small nests and cords of cells and single cells
- Eosinophilic to clear cytoplasm
- Ill-defined cytoplasmic borders

- Uniform round to oval nuclei
- Occasional spindled to serpentine nuclei
- Bland nuclear features
- Pleomorphism and atypia (rare)
- Mitoses (variable)
- Abundant fibromyxoid matrix
- Chondroid metaplasia (variable)
- Osteoid (rare)

DIFFERENTIAL DIAGNOSIS

- Neurofibroma
- Cutaneous mixed (adnexal/myoepithelial) tumor
- Extraskeletal myxoid chondrosarcoma

- Malignant peripheral nerve sheath tumor
- Extraskeletal osteosarcoma

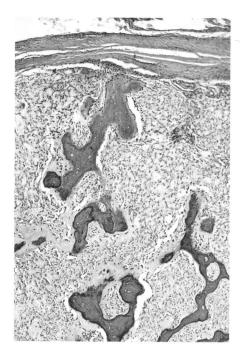

Fig. 14-17 An ossifying fibromyxoid tumor of soft parts in which the spicules of bone are perpendicular to the fibrous capsule.

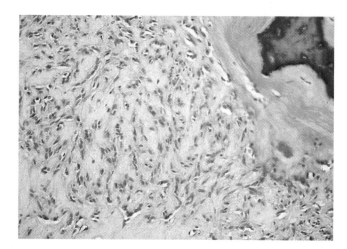

Fig. 14-18 A case of ossifying fibromyxoid tumor of soft parts demonstrating a peripheral rim of lamellar bone.

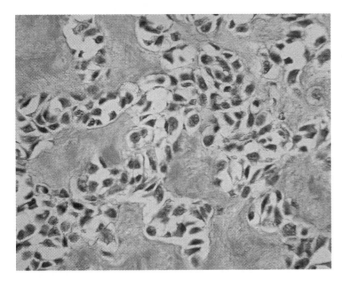

Fig. 14-19 An ossifying fibromyxoid tumor with a prominent hyalinized matrix.

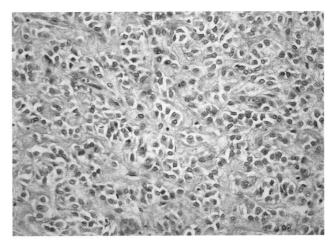

Fig. 14-20 A case of ossifying fibromyxoid tumor of soft parts with increased cellularity.

MALIGNANT

Alveolar Soft Part Sarcoma

Alveolar soft part sarcoma is rare and accounts for less than 1% of all soft tissue sarcomas. It occurs chiefly in adolescents and young adults and more commonly in females. Tumors in adults tend to involve the lower extremities, particularly the thigh, whereas those in children tend to involve the head and neck, especially the periorbital region and the tongue. Like many other sarcomas, it is slowly growing and usually painless. Patients present with distant metastases in one third of cases; these are usually to the lungs or brain. Prognosis is bleak; roughly 60% of patients are alive at 5 years and 45% to 50% at 10 years despite radical surgery and adjuvant therapy. Metastases are most frequently to the lungs, brain, and bone and rarely to lymph nodes. Children tend to have a more favorable prognosis, probably due to smaller tumors. The histogenesis is uncertain; the preponderance of immunohistochemical evidence suggests skeletal muscle differentiation, although theses results are inconclusive. The precise content of the characteristic intracytoplasmic crystals is unknown.

MICROSCOPIC FEATURES

- Relatively well circumscribed
- Fibrous septa
- Organoid growth pattern with nests and islands of cells
- Pseudoalveolar pattern due to loss of cellular cohesion (centrally)
- Sheetlike growth pattern with smaller cells (variable, primarily in children)
- Polygonal cells with abundant, granular, eosinophilic cytoplasm
- Clear cytoplasm (variable)

- Intracytoplasmic crystals (PAS +, diastase resistant)
- Intracytoplasmic glycogen
- Relatively uniform cells
- Pleomorphic cells (rare)
- Mitoses (rare)
- Rich, delicate, sinusoidal-like vasculature investing nests of cells
- Dilated, large veins at periphery of lesion
- Vascular invasion
- Fibrosis (variable)

DIFFERENTIAL DIAGNOSIS

- Renal cell carcinoma
- Melanoma
- Paraganglioma

- Granular cell tumor
- Rhabdomyosarcoma

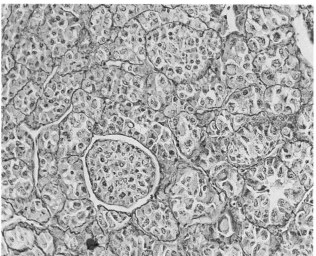

14-21

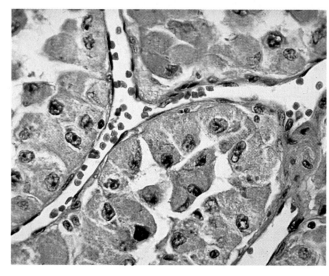

14-22

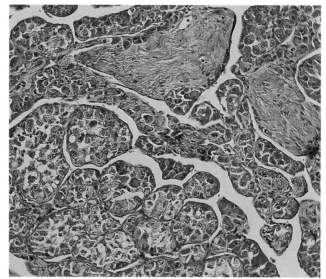

14-23

Figs. 14-21 through 14-23 Various examples of alveolar soft part sarcoma demonstrating distinct nests of cells surrounded by a delicate, inconpicuous, thin-walled vasculature. Centrally, the cells within the nested areas are discohesive and consequently have an alveolar appearance. The constituent cells usually have abundant, eosinophilic, granular cytoplasm, although clear cytoplasm may also be seen. Intracytoplasmic crystals may be seen in some hematoxylin-eosin stained sections. (Fig. 14-23, trichrome stain).

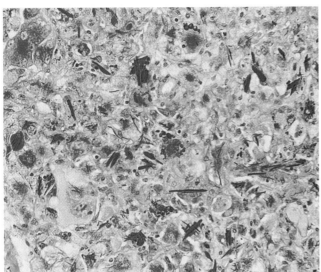

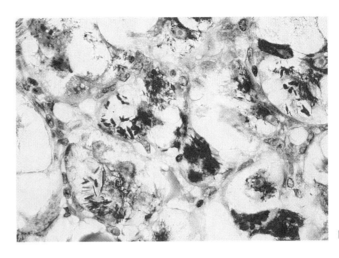

Figs. 14-24 and 14-25 PAS stains with diastase digestion unmask numerous and characteristic cytoplasmic crystals in these examples of alveolar soft part sarcoma.

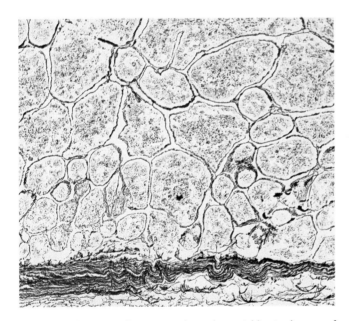

Fig. 14-26 The reticulin stain outlines the variably sized nests of alveolar soft part sarcoma.

Epithelioid Sarcoma

Epithelioid sarcoma occurs predominantly in the distal extremities of young adults, particularly in the fingers, hands, and forearm. It is characterized by a slow, relentless course with multiple local recurrences, eventual metastases, and death despite radical surgery and adjuvant therapy. It may involve the dermis, subcutis, fascia, or tendons as either a solitary or multinodular painless mass. The extent of tumor is frequently underestimated both clinically and pathologically due to insidious growth along fascial planes and merging with non-lesional fibroblasts. Long-term follow-up reveals a metastatic rate of approximately 50%, chiefly to lungs, followed by lymph nodes, skin and soft tissue, and the central nervous system. The prognosis is related to tumor site, size, depth, mitotic rate, necrosis, and vascular invasion, although which if any of these factors are independent variables is unknown.

MICROSCOPIC FEATURES

- Relatively circumscribed
- Multinodular or coalescing nodules simulating granulomas
- Central degeneration (loss of cellular cohesion) and necrosis
- Polygonal to spindle-shaped cells
- Deeply acidophilic, glassy cytoplasm (epithelioid cells)
- Eosinophilic to clear cytoplasm (spindle cells)
- Cytoplasmic vacuoles simulating vascular lumina (rare)

- Relatively uniform cells
- Multinucleated tumor cells (rare)
- Extensive hyalinization
- Chronic inflammation surrounding tumor
- Bone or calcification (rare)
- Cartilage (rare)
- Hemorrhage and cystic change (variable)
- Vascular invasion

DIFFERENTIAL DIAGNOSIS

- Infectious or necrobiotic granuloma
- Fibromatosis
- Nodular fasciitis
- Fibrous histiocytoma
- Squamous carcinoma
- Synovial sarcoma
- Epithelioid hemangioendothelioma
- Epithelioid angiosarcoma

- Mesothelioma
- Melanoma
- Fibrosarcoma
- Malignant fibrous histiocytoma
- Extraskeletal osteosarcoma
- Extrarenal rhabdoid tumor
- Rhabdomyosarcoma

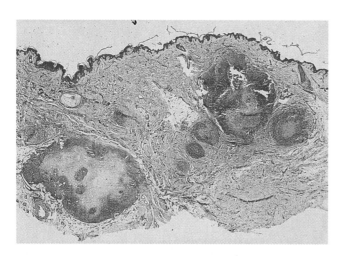

Fig. 14-27 Low magnification of epithelioid sarcoma showing primarily involvement of the skin, subcutis, and underlying fibrous connective tissue as multiple discrete to coalescing nodules, with centrally necrotic zones resulting in a granulomatous appearance.

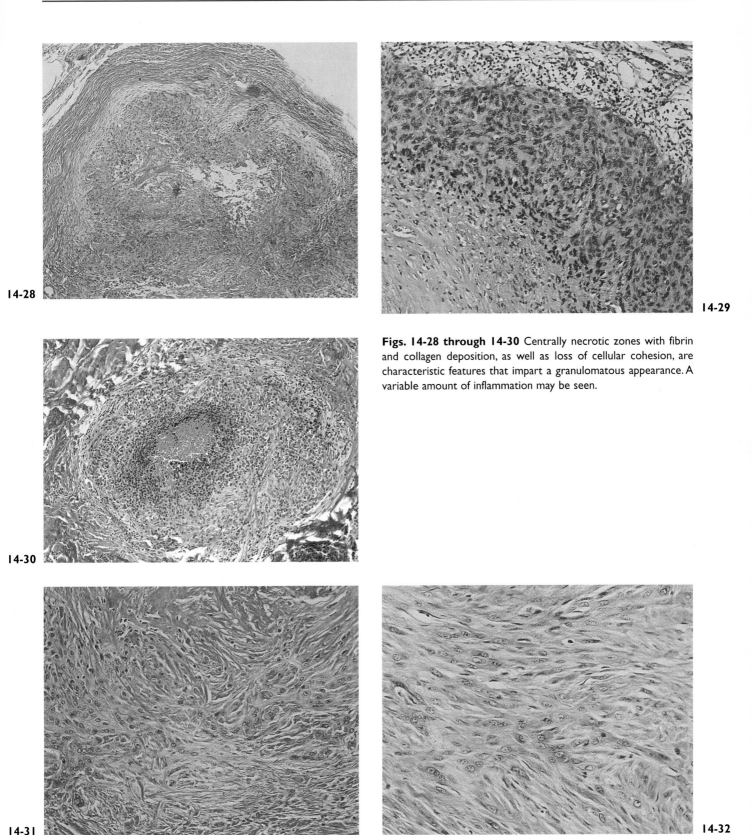

14-28

14-29

Figs. 14-28 through 14-30 Centrally necrotic zones with fibrin and collagen deposition, as well as loss of cellular cohesion, are characteristic features that impart a granulomatous appearance. A variable amount of inflammation may be seen.

14-30

14-31

14-32

Figs. 14-31 and 14-32 Spindled cells with clear to eosinophilic cytoplasm associated with collagen deposition cause epithelioid sarcoma to be confused with fibroblastic lesions. Both epithelioid and spindle cell zones may be seen in the same lesion.

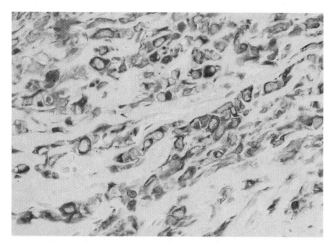

Fig. 14-33 Immunohistochemical stains for cytokeratin and vimentin are typically diffusely and strongly positive in both the epithelioid and spindle cell components of epithelioid sarcoma (cytokeratin immunostain).

Extraskeletal Ewing's Sarcoma

The histogenesis of extraskeletal Ewing's sarcoma is controversial. Some believe it is a neoplasm of primitive mesenchymal cells. Others believe that it is closely related to Ewing's sarcoma of bone and primitive neuroectodermal tumor/peripheral neuroepithelioma because of similar chromosomal aberrations, tissue culture properties, and immunohistochemical profiles (see discussion of primitive neuroectodermal tumor/peripheral neuroepithelioma). Extraskeletal Ewing's sarcoma is a tumor of adolescents and young adults that occurs primarily in the paravertebral regions, chest wall, retroperitoneum, and lower extremities. It grows rapidly and is associated with pain in one third of cases. Treatment is similar to Ewing's sarcoma of bone, with excision followed by radiation and chemotherapy. Metastases are common and primarily to the lungs and bone; lymph node metastases are rare. Late recurrences and involvement of the central nervous system may be seen. Necrosis is an important prognostic factor. Secondary sarcomas may supervene several years after radiation therapy.

MICROSCOPIC FEATURES

- Sheets of cells with a vaguely lobular pattern
- Pseudorosettes (rare)
- Uniform, monotonous, round cells
- Scant, clear, ill-defined cytoplasm
- Intracytoplasmic glycogen
- Finely dispersed chromatin and small nucleoli
- Pleomorphism (rare)
- Mitoses (variable)
- Crushed, necrotic cells resulting in a "filigreed" pattern
- Rich, delicate, inconspicuous vasculature
- Reticulin-poor matrix

DIFFERENTIAL DIAGNOSIS

- Ewing's sarcoma of bone
- Peripheral neuroepithelioma
- Neuroblastoma
- Neuroendocrine carcinoma (Merkel cell, small cell carcinoma of lung)
- Melanoma
- Lymphoma
- Granulocytic sarcoma
- Rhabdomyosarcoma
- Small cell osteosarcoma
- Hemangiopericytoma
- Angiosarcoma

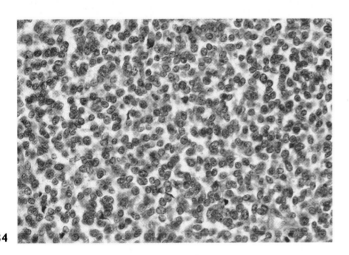

14-34

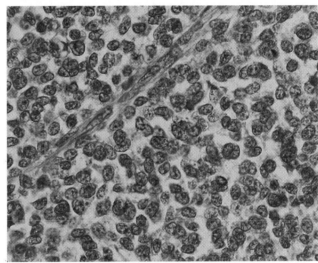

14-35

Figs. 14-34 and 14-35 Examples of extraskeletal Ewing's sarcoma demonstrating a highly cellular tumor composed of small, round, uniform cells with scant, clear cytoplasm and a finely distributed chromatin pattern.

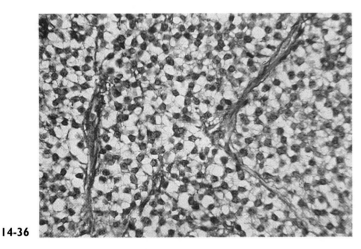

14-36

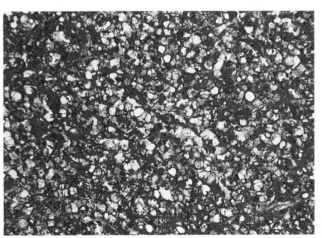

14-37

Figs. 14-36 and 14-37 A case of extraskeletal Ewing's sarcoma with a moderate amount of clear cytoplasm containing abundant glycogen. (PAS stain, Fig. 14-37. Figs 14-36 and 14-37 are the same case.)

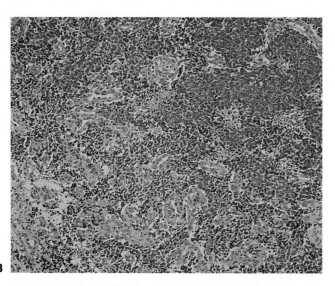

14-38

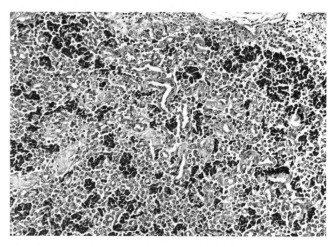

14-39

Figs. 14-38 and 14-39 Crushed, necrotic cells (filigree pattern) are seen in these cases of extraskeletal Ewing's sarcoma.

Extrarenal Rhabdoid Tumor

This rare and rather ill-defined malignant neoplasm tends to occur in infants and young children and less frequently in adolescents and adults. Rhaboid tumor was first recognized in the kidney when it was discovered to be distinct from Wilms' tumor. Those cases occurring outside the kidney are histologically similar and may involve virtually any site. Their relationship, if any, to renal rhabdoid tumor is unclear. Rare multicentric rhabdoid tumors may occur. Rhabdoid tumors of soft tissue tend to involve the trunk and proximal extremities and are typically deep seated, although the subcutis and skin may be secondarily involved. Metastases are usually to lungs, liver, lymph nodes, and other soft tissue sites. They are extremely aggressive and recalcitrant to therapy; median survival in a relatively large series of soft tissue rhabdoid tumors was 6 months. Consistent chromosomal abnormalities have not been identified. The distinctive histologic appearance of the tumor is primarily attributable to the presence of abundant intracytoplasmic whorls of intermediate filaments that stain for vimentin and keratin. Some investigators have postulated that rhabdoid tumors arise from primitive, pluripotential mesenchymal cells that have the ability to express epithelial and mesenchymal markers. Others contend that it is merely a malignant neoplasm that may represent either a nonspecific or high-grade, end-stage phenotype, somewhat analagous to "dedifferentiated" sarcomas.

MICROSCOPIC FEATURES

- Infiltrative, destructive growth pattern
- Solid to discohesive sheets of cells or trabeculae
- Scant basophilic to amphophilic cytoplasm
- Prominent, amorphous, paranuclear, eosinophilic globules (corresponding to intermediate filaments)

- Large, vesicular, round to reniform nuclei
- Inclusion-like nucleoli, basophilic or eosinophilic
- Mitoses
- Necrosis

DIFFERENTIAL DIAGNOSIS

- Rhabdomyosarcoma
- Desmoplastic small round cell tumor of infancy and childhood
- Epithelioid sarcoma

- Primitive, epithelioid malignant schwannoma
- Melanoma
- Poorly differentiated carcinoma

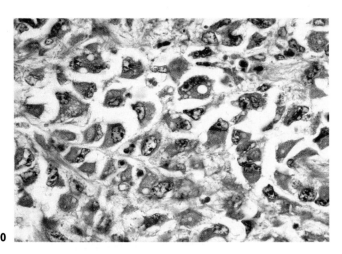
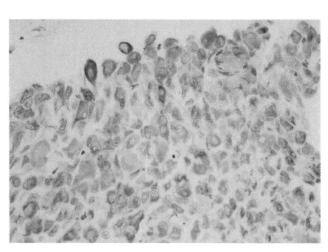

14-40   14-41

Figs. 14-40 and 14-41 A case of extrarenal rhabdoid tumor of soft tissue in which the cells are arranged in sheets and have abundant, deeply acidophilic cytoplasm, vesicular nuclei, and prominent inclusion-like nucleoli. These lesions frequently express keratin (cytokeratin immunostain, Fig. 14-41).

Index

Vascular tumors
  benign, 138-159
  borderline, 159-163
  malignant, 164-170
Venous hemangioma, 139
von Recklinghausen's disease, 221, 222, 224, 234-235

W

Well-differentiated extraskeletal chondrosarcoma, 265
Well-differentiated liposarcoma, 93, 94-98

Well-differentiated papillary mesothelioma, 205-206
Wilms' tumor, 296

X

Xanthogranuloma, juvenile, 51-52
Xanthoma, 53-54
Xanthomatous malignant fibrous histiocytoma, 71